Nursing Care of the
Adult Urology Patient

Nursing Care of the
Adult Urology Patient

Sylvia L. Whitehead, R.N., Ed.M.
Coordinator of Educational Delineation
School of Nursing, University of Hawaii:
Formerly *Instructor, Department of Surgery,*
St. Vincent's Hospital and Medical Center of New York.

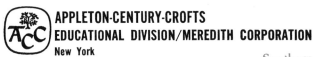

APPLETON-CENTURY-CROFTS
EDUCATIONAL DIVISION/MEREDITH CORPORATION
New York

Copyright © 1970 by MEREDITH CORPORATION

760-1

Library of Congress Catalog Card Number: 70-109162

PRINTED IN THE UNITED STATES OF AMERICA
390-93690-1

To my husband, GERALD A. SUMIDA,
with appreciation for his encouragement and understanding.

Acknowledgments

My teaching experiences at the School of Nursing, St. Vincent's Hospital and Medical Center of New York, contributed substantially to the choice of material that has been included in this book. Special thanks are expressed for the guidance received from Sr. Mary Brigida who was Chairman of the Surgical Department during the time of my initial teaching venture and to Sr. Mary Robert, Director of the school, for her assistance and encouragement during the preparation of the manuscript.

Grateful acknowledgment is given to Miss Adele Spiegler, Medical Illustrator, for her untiring efforts in my behalf, and to Mr. Charles F. Bollinger, Editor-in-Chief, Nursing Education Department, Appleton-Century-Crofts, for his encouragement and support during those periods when I doubted that the manuscript would ever be completed. Special appreciation is expressed to Dr. Andrew J. McGowan, Jr., Chief, Division of Urology, Department of Surgery, St. Vincent's Hospital and Medical Center, Miss Eileen L. Kullman, R.N., Head Nurse of the Urologic Unit, and Mrs. Kathryn Parmelli Feeney, R.N., M.A., for their generosity in reading the manuscript, offering suggestions, and exchanging ideas about different approaches to the care of patients with urologic disorders. Sincere gratitude is also extended to Mrs. Nanette Schiff who typed the manuscript.

Warmest thanks are also expressed to the Freshmen of Entryway Six, Branford College, Yale University (1969), who provided so many hours of pleasant diversion and cheerful encouragement during the preparation of the manuscript.

Preface

At some time during the course of their education, student nurses will study and acquire clinical experience in caring for patients with diseases of the urogenital tract. The student will be expected to understand the dynamics of the physiologic processes which initiate urologic symptoms and to develop and implement nursing care plans specifically for the care of these patients. Therefore, this textbook has been written to provide a concise and explicit reference for students to facilitate their studies of the responsibilities of the nurse to the urologic patient. It is also the author's intention to foster the student's ability to conceptualize the dynamics of disease processes and the essentials of related nursing care so that a problem-solving orientation will be applied when nursing care is planned.

Only those disorders occurring in the adult male patient are stressed because the nursing care of adult female patients with genital disorders often comes within the province of gynecology and obstetrics, and is usually discussed at length in textbooks dealing with that subject matter. In like manner, care of children with urologic disorders is not elaborated because of the wealth of material available in pediatric textbooks. The scope of material presented is limited to the detailed examination of only those types of urogenital disorders that are encountered most frequently in the clinical situation: care of the patient with a urinary tract infection, renal calculi, benign prostatic hypertrophy, cancer of the prostate, cancer of the kidney, and cancer of the bladder. Care of the patient with testicular carcinoma and with tuberculosis of the kidney is also included because available literature on these subjects is limited and inadequate for the needs of nurses. The probability of encountering these uncommon disorders does increase, however, in urban institutions and in military hospitals where large numbers of young male patients receive medical assistance.

The first three chapters of the text (which include an overview of the principles of nursing care of patients with urologic disorders, the types and functions of equipment most frequently utilized on urologic units, and review of the anatomy and physiology of the urinary system) provide the general framework upon which differentiated aspects of nursing care on a urologic unit are progressively superimposed. Although the book has been written with the assumption that the student has acquired basic knowledge of normal anatomy and physiology, and of the general principles of medical and surgical nursing prior to receiving clinical experience in urology, review sections are incorporated within the chapters to facilitate recall as disease processes of specific structures are presented.

Special treatment is given to the introduction of urologic terminology. Category-set principles—a technique adapted from mathematical set theory—and etymologic approaches to the understanding of new terms are elaborated in lieu of the utilization of traditional methods of definition. It is hoped that these modalities will stimulate the student to analyze new terminology when it is encountered. Another technique employed to encourage conscientious application of knowledge acquired by the student is the inclusion of patient-care studies at the end of selected chapters. Whenever assimilation of the numerous aspects of nursing care would tend to pose difficulty for the student, or whenever it seemed desirable to emphasize the operational steps involved in a problem-solving approach to patient care, these studies are presented. Specific modifications of care which are indicated when medical disorders complicate the general condition of the urologic patient or when postoperative complications may occur have also been interjected. In addition to the aforementioned innovative approaches to the teaching of nursing students, detailed explanations of treatments performed to accomplish the diagnostic work-up of the urologic patient are presented within the context of the disorder under investigation. Consequently, a chapter dealing with the enumeration and explanation of urologic diagnostic tests has been rendered unnecessary by this integrative method of presentation. This approach has proven helpful in encouraging the student to remember specific nursing care responsibilities related to patient needs prior to, during, and after such procedures.

Throughout the text, simple detailed explanations are used to clarify those types of processes or situations which tend to bewilder students during their urologic experience. It is hoped that the emphasis placed on patient-observation, the development and supervision of the nursing care plan, and patient-teaching will help the student define the unique role of the professional nurse on the urologic unit.

The references included at the end of each chapter represent those sources which are within the nurses realm of understanding and which are pertinent to sound nursing practice. Few references are dated earlier than 1963 because the ever-expanding scope of medical knowledge is constantly disproving or improving upon widely held theories and established practices.

Sylvia L. Whitehead

Contents

Nursing Care of the
Adult Urology Patient

1

The Nurse on the Urologic Unit

NURSE-PATIENT RELATIONSHIPS

It is often difficult to assign a parsimonious definition to the various divisions of medicine. However, simply stated, urology may be thought of as that specialized branch of medicine that is concerned with the urine and with diseases of the urogenital organs. Since care of the female patient who has disease or disorders of the reproductive tract comes within the scope of gynecology, that topic is not discussed in this text. However, care of the male patient who presents with genital-tract disease is discussed, as is the care of both male and female patients manifesting disease of the urinary tract.

The uniqueness of the contribution made by the nurse on a urologic unit lies in the functions formulated and implemented from role expectations with regard to specific situations arising on that unit. Major functions germane to the expertise of this nurse must be developed from innovative as well as established principles of sound nursing practice. Thus priorities for today's urologic nurse should include acquisition of knowledge regarding techniques of intervention which prevent the spread of infection, implementation of principles of rehabilitation which minimize dependency and assist the patient in realizing his maximum capabilities in spite of physical infirmity, and the coordination of the multiphasic services being rendered to the patient.

Inherent in this patient-oriented approach is the belief that (1) every person has equal rights to the highest standards of sound nursing practice; (2) the highest quality of care implies intervention measures appropriate to the needs of the person or persons involved; and (3) those in need must actively cooperate with the course of treatment being undertaken. Both verbal and nonverbal interaction characterizes the dynamic nurse-patient relationship. Both the nurse and the patient have psychologic needs, feelings, and a personal code of living. It should also be remembered that individuals strive to satisfy their own needs during episodes of interaction. Whenever an interaction occurs, it is initiated by a need. The nurse has perceptions of the role of a ministrant, of the role of a patient, and of the patient's needs in the specific situation. It is usually after this initial evaluation that the nurse conceptualizes the care required to satisfy the patient's needs. However, the patient also has perceptions of his situation and of the role of the nurse in relation to his needs. Thus the quality of the interpersonal relationship is an important aspect of the care and cure of the patient. Although both individuals have power, in the long run it is the patient who controls the outcome of the situation. The nurse may minister, counsel, instruct, encourage, and reassure, but it is the patient who must decide to cooperate and/or comply when the need arises.

There are many factors in the nurse-patient relationship which may act as barriers to appropriate nursing intervention. The nurse should realize that many patients feel that hospitalization robs them of identity and independence. It is difficult for these patients to accept help even though they are in need.

Other patients equate illness with punishment. Because such patients primarily tend to seek sympathy and emotional support, they often set up barriers to care directed toward cure and/or rehabilitation. Still others feel that their needs are so complex and unique that only the doctor is qualified to render care. On the other hand, nurses feel competent and a defensive, fearful patient is often perceived as being either resistive or uncooperative. Efforts by the nurse to counter this behavior often takes the form of arguing or pressuring of the patient in an attempt to obtain compliance. This in turn is usually met with more resistance and a deadlock results. Therefore, in establishing rapport, the nurse should strive to display behavior which will encourage trust and confidence so that the patient is encouraged to believe that "getting well" is a joint venture. If the patient continues to exhibit defensive, fearful, or dejected behavior, the nurse must accept him as he is and, if necessary, compromise in certain situations in order to meet his needs until such time as a change in behavior occurs.

To this end, the nurse should encourage opportunities for the gradual resumption of independence; the nature and manner of implementing this deserves consideration. By evaluating the patient's level of capability and by estimating his potential, the nurse develops a concept of possible target goals. Self-care activities may be planned and carried out thereafter. However, the nurse should remember that frustration occurs when an individual is asked to perform an independent activity which he cannot complete without assistance. The dejected patient, for example, often lacks the energy to execute even minimal amounts of self-care and his state of dejection deepens with failure. During the course of rendering care, the nurse should afford the patient the opportunity of achieving success in performing those aspects of care which are within his scope of management. This supportive technique exemplifies a form of tension-reducing intervention. Achievements of the patient should always be recorded in the nurses notes *and* on the nursing-care plan so that consistency of approach and gradual resumption of independence will be achieved. The nurse should also strive to make the patient feel better about his appearance because this is another step in helping him to regain a secure feeling of "self" and of personal worth. A man tends to feel sick if he is allowed to remain unshaven for days. A woman experiences the same feeling when her hair has not been combed for days. Poor grooming reinforces the patient's feelings of weakness and illness, regardless of his rate of medical progress.

THE NURSE'S ROLES

It seems clear then that the nurse on the urologic unit has two roles: administrative and ministrative. Knowledge of and skills in the clinical aspects of urologic treatment qualify this professional for a ministrative (providing care or aid) role. Knowledge of the principles underlying the medical aspects of specific disease entities—as well as related social and psychologic factors implicit in human behavior—qualify this professional for an administrative or management role. The professional nurse on the urologic unit is qualified for the planning, coordination, and evaluation of nursing services rendered to meet the patient's needs. It is true, however, that these are roles that the nurse has assumed in other settings. Taking this into consideration, it may be concluded that these roles are *not unique* to the expertise of the nurse on the urologic unit. Therefore, the uniqueness of this nurse must lie either in the functions performed in the execution of these roles or in the manner of their implementation (see Fig. 1). The major functions listed in the diagram are conceptual delineations, and the professional nurse on the urologic unit (as a member of a health team) will be able to execute them only to that degree consonant with a particular clinical situation.

A function involves action or activity to accomplish goal-

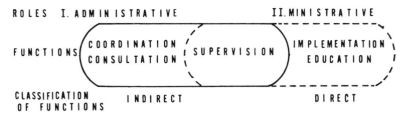

ROLES   I. ADMINISTRATIVE   II. MINISTRATIVE

FUNCTIONS COORDINATION SUPERVISION   IMPLEMENTATION
           CONSULTATION   EDUCATION

CLASSIFICATION   INDIRECT   DIRECT
OF FUNCTIONS

Fig. 1. Schematic diagram of the roles and major functions of the professional nurse on a urologic unit.

directed objectives and—in an interactional situation—actions carried out in a patterned sequence may be considered as functions of a specific role. The administrative role implies directing or managing; two of the main functions executed by the urologic-unit nurse are coordination and consultation. Coordination involves the ordering and/or interrelating of the medical aspects of patient services, as well as participation in the planning and development of the nursing-care plan. Consultation involves the providing of resource services for other nurses of the staff and to administrators. An indirect classification is given to these functions because there is no direct interaction between the nurse and the patients being served. However, the coordinator and/or consultant may have contact with persons who will in turn provide direct services to these patients.

The *ministrative* role includes care or tending; its functions are considered to be "direct" because there is unmediated interaction between the nurse and the patient or patient-delivery systems. Education is a central focus of the ministrative role of the professional nurse; this nurse often participates in individual as well as family counseling, and may even instruct groups of patients. Information is imparted about the promotion and maintenance of good health, the prevention of urogenital infections, and/or the rehabilitative aspects of patient care. Because interpretation is an essential function of this role, the nurse often acts as liaison between the patient and the doctor as well as between the patient and his family. The implementation aspect of the ministrative role is a recurrent theme of the text and is elaborated in a general manner later in this chapter.

The remaining major function—supervision—seems to

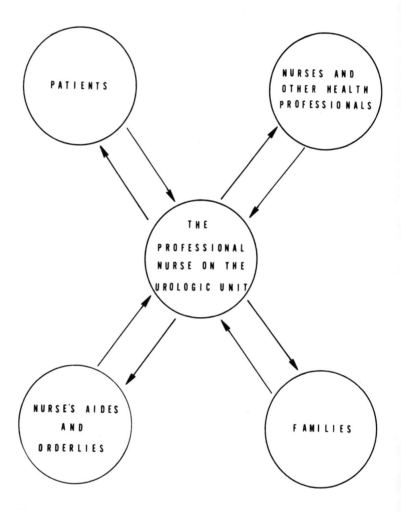

Fig. 2. Schematic representation of the major service interactions of the professional nurse on the urologic unit.

have administrative *and* ministrative aspects. Administrative aspects of supervision are concerned with the instructing of aides toward increasing their effectiveness when they render services to patients. The supervisor emphasizes the application of principles of rehabilitation and approaches to changed behavior, as well as the dynamics of behavioral changes caused by the stress of illness. The supervisor in this situation is also concerned with the orientation of new professional nurses and with the observation and direction of intervention measures employed by staff nurses and nurse's aides. Ministrative aspects of supervision are concerned with observation and guidance during the interval when patients are learning self-care.

Thus the uniqueness of the nurse on a urologic unit is dependent upon the extent to which this professional is allowed to implement the functions discussed and in the individual attributes of the particular nurse. The functional relationships of the urologic-unit nurse are diagrammatically represented in Figure 2.

THE UROLOGIC-UNIT PATIENT

The nurse working on a urologic unit will observe that the patients are predominantly in the older age group, and she should be aware that hospitalization is an especially anxiety-evoking experience for them. Thoughts of death and fear of cancer are usually the primary sources of much of the apprehension which is manifested, but the overriding question (which may or may not be verbalized) is whether he is being told the truth about his condition. To compound matters, patients in the older age group often have an associated disease which complicates the urologic symptoms; it must also be remembered that the general physical condition of the patient may present unanticipated problems. When all these considerations are evaluated, the nurse should be able to appreciate how superficial and inadequate some phrases—such as "Don't you worry now" and "Everything is going to be all right"—are when used in efforts to comfort these patients. False assurances are actually insulting to the patient's intelligence. A reality-oriented approach is superior because it fosters the patient's ability to cope with his situation. Words of reassurance to urologic patients are best triggered by what the patients say. The nurse should allow such patients to express their thoughts and feelings—however uncomfortable this may be for the listener—and then try to allay apprehensions by assisting patients to find appropriate solutions to problems as they arise.

Unfamiliar surroundings are initially threatening to many individuals and are most certainly threatening to the elderly, who tend to reminisce and cling to those things that are familiar. Often a brief orientation to the unit, followed by an introduction to another patient who is sociable, will make the period of adjustment less difficult. A cheerful, pleasant approach should be employed when one cares for the urologic patient, but adequate quiet must be afforded these patients because rest is especially important to their recovery. The individual patient cubicle as well as the entire unit should be adequately ventilated and urinary drainage should be emptied frequently. Gone are the days when a urologic unit could be identified by the smell! The nurse should allow no more than 500 ml of urine to collect in a drainage receptacle at any given time, and prompt emptying of urinals used by patients on bed rest will also help to eliminate odor.

Many of the patients will need assistance with or supervision of their daily bath; and, although this may not be requested, the nurse should volunteer such assistance. When bed baths are taken, the washing of the back and legs may pose a problem. In this instance a positive approach, "Let me wash your back for you; I know it's difficult to reach back there," rather than a questioning one, "Do you need any help?" is most effective in securing the desired result: a refreshed patient.

Since a shower or tub bath is usually more satisfying and effective than what can be achieved with a basin provided at the bedside, the nurse should try to obtain such an order from the doctor when it seems feasible and such facilities are available. For older patients who may have difficulty standing in a shower, a straight-backed chair may be provided so that they can sit while washing. Others may need assistance in getting in and out of the tub, but they should be afforded privacy during their bath once they are in the tub. After they are helped out of the tub, privacy may again be allowed during the drying-off period by placing a chair for the patient to sit on in the tub room. Allowing the patient to do as much for himself as he can (and as much as safety standards will allow) by giving assistance only when indicated minimizes his feelings of dependency and helplessness.

Ambulation should be encouraged since many patients in the older age group have circulatory problems secondary to vascular changes. Such problems make bedrest undesirable unless it is specifically ordered or indicated as part of the prescribed treatment of a patient. It must also be remembered that inactivity may result in respiratory as well as circulatory complications. Thus gentle but firm encouragement should be used to keep such patients mobile. Again, a questioning approach should be avoided; the nurse who asks the urologic patient if he's ready to get out of bed will either be answered negatively or will encourage procrastination. While a foot stool is being moved to the side of the bed or while the head of the bed is being slowly elevated so that the patient will be in a better position to manuever himself into an upright position, the nurse can make a simple statement about assisting him to get up. This positive approach has proved to be most effective.

Those patients who are embarrassed by their drainage apparatus may be encouraged to ambulate if the nurse places a hand towel over the drainage bag. The nurse should also instruct the patient to hold the drainage receptacle lower than bladder level as he is walking and lower than chair-seat level when he is sitting. Unless forewarned and supervised periodically thereafter, patients with indwelling catheters and drainage receptacles tend to hold the receptacle waist high as they walk or to place it on their laps when they are seated. This is to be discouraged because drainage of urine becomes sluggish and retention is encouraged. Patients should also be taught to elevate the distal part of the drainage tubing from time to time so that urine flows into the collecting receptacle and does not remain trapped in the tubing. The lower part of the tubing often loops down below the drainage bag, causing an anti-gravity flow—urine must move uphill to reach the collecting receptacle. Concurrently, the urine backs up in the tubing, which results in sluggish outflow and stasis in the bladder.

Diet and fluid intake and output are important considerations in the care of the urologic patient. Maintaining or improving the patient's general physical status is crucial to his recovery. The ingestion of large amounts of fluid to accomplish the "physiologic irrigation" of the urinary tract is a tenet of urologic management. The elderly tend to eat infrequently and in small amounts, and to drink little fluid generally. Therefore, the nurse may have to assist at mealtime in order to encourage the patient to eat, and to see that fluids are taken at regular intervals during the day. Assistance at mealtime should include positioning of the patient *before* the meal is served, so that his physiologic alignment with and proximity to the table on which the food tray is to be placed do not inhibit his eating. The nurse should also refrain from rushing the patient through the meal. Some patients, of course, will procrastinate and limits must be set, but this can be accomplished short of "shoveling" food into the patient's mouth or arguing with him about his minimal intake. Such strategies as the best approach to be utilized in facilitating implementation of care, as well as other cues that will assist in coping with the individual's personality should be included in the nursing-care plan. When such information is shared with and/or made available to other members of the nursing team, time is saved during the staff-patient rapport stage of hospitalization, and nursing care is expedited. Being busy and experiencing the tension that limited time schedules impose are the nature of things in nursing, and all nurses must come to terms with this as part of their professional growth and development. To impose these burdens on patients—at any time—may result in the relief of tension for the nurse, but such an imposition results in additional stress for the patient. These episodes, therefore, are definitely to be avoided at mealtime.

In addition to the aforementioned suggestions, the nurse should make an attempt to ascertain the food preferences of the urologic patient. Among the foods permitted within the limitations of his particular diet, the patient will often have preferences which he will neglect to request from the dietary service; the nurse can be a most effective liaison between the patient and the dietician in such instances. By finding out which foods and beverages the patient likes best and then notifying the dietician of these preferences, the nurse helps to provide a choice from a variety of foods which the patient will consider palatable. Through this process, the nurse may be indirectly encouraging the patient to eat. A regular diet is generally ordered for the urologic patient—unless some associated disease, such as diabetes or a cardiac condition, precludes its use.

The desired oral fluid intake of most urologic patients is between 2,500 and 4,000 ml per day. This gives the nurse the mandate to force fluids on the patients. Most of this total daily fluid intake should be taken during the day and evening hours so that frequency of urination does not inordinately disturb the patient's sleep. An 8-ounce glass of water (or other beverage) each hour during the suggested time interval will accomplish the intake goal.

It should be mentioned at this juncture that patients—regardless of age group—generally find it difficult to drink all of the contents of an 8-ounce glass of fluid at any given time. It should also be particularly noted that older patients *normally* tend to restrict their fluid intake, and therefore require the utilization of special management strategy. The urologic-unit nurse who is attempting to force fluids should remember that liquids served at room temperature are usually tolerated better than iced liquids. Water in large amounts is ordinarily not palatable for the patient, but—by alternating water with other fluids such as fruit juices, tea, coffee, broth, or milk—the nurse can provide the patient with a tastier variety and make the assignment of forcing fluids less problematic. The nurse will also observe that *two* 4-ounce glasses of fluid will be ingested more readily than one 8-ounce glass. The truly enterprising nurse will offer one half-filled, 8-ounce glass of fluid to the patient and follow that approximately half an hour later with another half-filled 8-ounce glass. Since time is such a relative dimension for hospitalized people, patients usually cooperate because they feel that a concession has been made. By offering liquids in this manner, the nurse tends to accomplish the objective of forcing fluids.

In many instances, a quantitative measure of urinary output is also an important aspect of patient care. When large amounts of fluid are ingested, the nurse must be alert to the possibility of retention and its inherent consequences: extreme discomfort for the patient and the potential for infection. Although professional and ancillary personnel endeavor to keep accurate records of intake and output when requested to do so, it has been found that teaching the patient is the most valuable key to precise recording. Therefore, the nurse would do well to explain to the patient, whenever feasible, that accurate recording of intake and output is essential to the planning of his course of treatment. Then a slip of paper should be provided at the bedside as a worksheet (see Fig. 3) or an "intake" and "output" form may be used if available. The important factor in this instance is ease of accessibility for the patient's recording efforts.

INTAKE		OUTPUT	
Time	**Amount**	**Time**	**Amount**
8–12 N	~~LHT~~ ~~LHT~~ ////	8 AM	200 U
		9:15 AM	200 U
		10:45 AM	250 U
		11:50 AM	150 U
12N–4PM	~~LHT~~ ~~LHT~~ //	2 PM	350 U
		3 PM	160 E
4PM–8PM	~~LHT~~ ~~LHT~~	4:15 PM	210 U
		5:30 PM	200 U
		6:45 PM	300 U
8PM–Mn	~~LHT~~ ~~LHT~~	7:30 PM	150 U
		8:15 PM	200 U
		10 PM	180 U
Mn–8AM	~~LHT~~ /	2 AM	200 U
		6 AM	210 U
24 Hour	Total (52 × 60) 3120 cc	24 Hour Total	2800 U 160 E

Name: J. Fortell   Date: 10/17

NB: Each tally mark= 60cc; U=urine; E=emesis; Time of each voiding should be recorded

Fig. 3. An intake and output worksheet. A slip of paper may be left at the patient's bedside for the recording of intake and output. The patient places a tally stroke in the intake column each time he drinks a glass of fluid. Each tally stroke represents 60 ml of fluid. To calculate the total fluid intake, the nurse adds the tally strokes and multiplies the total by 60. (**U** under the output column represents urinary output; the **E** indicates an emesis.)

A graduated measuring receptacle for output may then be provided for the patient. Instruction should be given regarding the manner in which the graduations on the receptacle should be read, and some practice readings should be tried. If the patient is successful in the trial efforts, he should be allowed to record his output. If he is unsuccessful, he should be told to leave the urine in the urinal and should be reassured that the nurse will make rounds periodically to measure and dispose of his output.

All patients should be told when their urine is to be measured. Many will prefer to void in the bathroom and may be allowed to do so if they will void in a urinal and measure the amount before it is discarded. Some nurses on urologic units prefer to have patients void in a urinal (labeled with their name) and leave it in the utility room, when periodic checks are made. In this way the nurse may record the amount voided on a worksheet over the discard receptacle; the patient may pick up his urinal on the way to the bathroom each time he wants to void.

As for intake, a stack of 60-ml drinking cups may be provided and the patient should be instructed to drink liquids only from the cups provided. This will necessitate having liquids transferred from original containers to the cups stacked on the bedside table. The patient may then be taught to make a tally stroke on the intake and output worksheet (see Fig. 3) each time he drinks a cup of fluid. This method usually proves more accurate than trusting the patient to remember the amount of liquid contained in the various-sized receptacles that are received during the course of the day. This method is a more desirable approach to the accurate recording of intake than having the patient count the number of times the water pitcher has been filled during the day. The nurse will notice that half-filled water pitchers are often filled, or discarded and refilled, which causes inaccurate measurements of fluid intake. Warm liquids such as soup, tea, or coffee are usually served in 100- to 150-ml containers and the patient may be advised of this so he may record intake accordingly.

The patient should also be instructed to record fluids taken at mealtime immediately after the meal—while memory is fresh or while the tray is still available for verification if the patient is not reliable.

The nurse should also be aware of another characteristic of urologic patients: they often have irregular bowel habits or take laxatives regularly when at home. Thus constipation can be a management problem on a urologic unit. Scrupulous daily recording of the patient's bowel movements will aid the observant nurse is detecting this condition early. When this aspect of the gross physiologic functioning is overlooked in patients of the older age group particularly, impaction frequently occurs. Relief of this condition is effected through treatments which are extremely uncomfortable and tiring to these individuals. The nurse working with urologic patients would, therefore, do well to bring the question of constipation to the doctor's attention early so that PRN orders for cathartic may be written. It has been found that warm water added to half a glass of prune juice in the mornings or twice daily will tend to foster regularity. Hot water and lemon juice will often have a similar effect.

This overview of the care of the patient on a urologic unit will conclude with brief mention of the importance of observing vital signs. Instrumentation is a frequent occurrence for these patients and the possibility of mechanical trauma or bacterial invasion is great. Temperature spikes, therefore, are a significant index of inflammatory or infectious processes in the urinary tract and should be reported to the doctor promptly. The patient's temperature should always be taken as ordered.

For the patient who enters with hematuria, blood pressure readings and pulse rate are extremely important. These indices are usually taken periodically during the day in such cases because such a patient may go into shock. The nurse should be prepared for this eventuality by having necessary equipment on the unit which can be easily mobilized. The doctor must also be kept informed about the patient's progress and/or changes in vital signs.

REFERENCES

1. Basowitz, H., et al. Anxiety and Stress. New York, McGraw-Hill Book Company, 1955.
2. Francis, G. M. Cancer: the emotional component. Amer. J. Nurs., 69: 1677–81, 1969.

3.   Sarbin, T. R. Role theory. In Lindzey, G., ed. Handbook of Social Psychology. Reading, Mass., Addison-Wesley Publishing Co., Inc., Vol. 1, 1954.
4.   Selye, H. The Stress of Life. New York, McGraw-Hill Book Company, 1956.

2

The Urinary System

The most comprehensive way to begin the study of nursing care of the patient with urologic disease is through the pyramidal approach (see Fig. 1). After the student has acquired a working knowledge of the anatomy and physiology of the genitourinary system, later additions to these fundamentals will "click" on both thinking and doing levels—ultimately expressed in the nurse's care of patients.

Therefore, as a means of integrating previously learned facts into functional understanding, a review of the urinary system seems appropriate at this juncture. In this review section, an overview of renal circulation, neural control, and hormonal influence of the urinary system will be provided along with a discussion of the dynamics of micturition (urination). While working with a urologist, the student will often hear basic urinary-tract structures referred to by names other than the ones with which she is familiar; therefore, alternate terminology will also be introduced in this chapter (and used interchangeably) in efforts to keep confusion to a minimum.

17

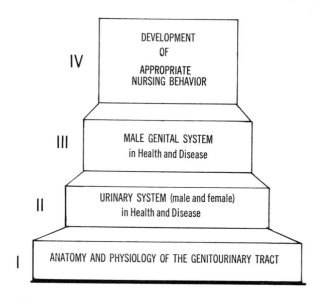

Fig. 1. Diagrammatic representation of the pyramidal approach to the study of nursing care of the patient with urologic disease. After the student has acquired a working knowledge of the anatomy and physiology of the genitourinary system (Step I), the way is paved for in-depth study of the urinary system and the male genital system which is so intimately integrated with it (Steps II and III respectively). The ultimate effect of this progression of ever-narrowing focus is the development of appropriate nursing behavior (Step IV).

An overview of the male reproductive system will be presented later in the text.

AN ANATOMIC REVIEW

When one considers the urinary system, four structures should come to mind: the kidneys, ureters, bladder, and urethra. *Renal* is a term often used when the kidney is referred to, and the term *vesical* is often used interchangeably for the bladder.

On gross inspection (see Fig. 2), the kidney is seen as an oblong, convex-concave-shaped organ which is from 10 to

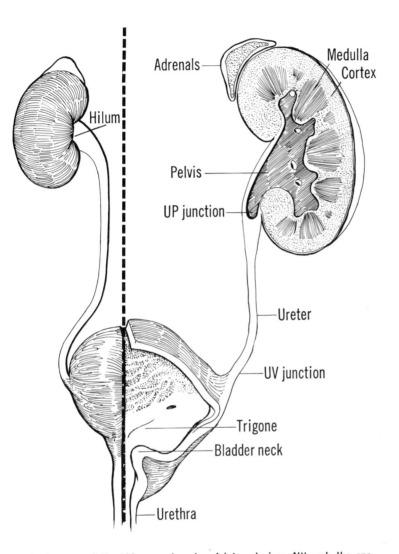

Fig. 2. Anatomy of the kidney—external and internal view. Although the anatomic position of the kidney has not been included, it should be remembered that the kidneys are located in the costovertebral angle (CVA) in the retroperitoneal position. The bladder, however, lies in a suprapubic position (above the pubic arch). The right kidney is usually a little lower than the left because of the large space occupied by the liver.

12 cm in length. It is composed of two layers: an outer *cortex* and an inner *medulla*. These two layers collectively are what is referred to as the *kidney parenchyma*: the essential part of the kidney, concerned specifically with function. Therefore, the term *parenchyma* distinguishes the functional part of the kidney from its connective tissue covering (the *renal capsule*). The renal pelvis, the ureters, and the bladder comprise the *collecting system* of the kidney. Terms pertaining to the kidney (or renal) pelvis often have the prefix *pyelo-*, while those referring to the kidney (or renal) parenchyma have the prefix *nephro-*.

It will further be noted that there are three physiologic narrowings in the urinary tract. The kidney pelvis has a normal capacity of from 8 to 10 ml, and the region where it narrows and elongates to become the ureter is commonly referred to as the *ureteropelvic junction*—the UP junction. The second narrowing in the tract occurs where the ureter enters the bladder (or vesical); this is referred to as the *ureterovesical junction*—the UV junction. The last narrowing occurs at the apex of the bladder, where the urethra is met. This is not called a junction, but is usually referred to by region only: the *bladder neck*. These physiologic narrowings become particularly important when calculus formation occurs. Stones may become lodged in any one of these areas and cause obstruction to the free flow of urine.

If imaginary lines were drawn within the bladder connecting the terminal openings of the two ureters and the urethra, a triangle would be formed—the *trigone*. The *tri-* in trigone, then, refers to the area near the base of the bladder where three openings may be observed: the area where the two ureters enter and the urethra exits.

In addition to knowing which structures comprise the urinary system, a knowledge of where they are located is also important. The angle formed by the attachment of the lower-most ribs to the vertebral column is called the costovertebral angle (the CVA—not to be confused with cerebrovascular accident). It is approximately at the level of the first lumbar vertebra, within the CVA, and in the retroperitoneal position (i.e., behind the peritoneal cavity) that the kidneys are to be found. Frequently a complaint of CVA tenderness is an important diagnostic aid, and kidney disease must be ruled out. The kidney parenchyma, kidney pelvis, and the upper portion of the ureter are located in this area. The ureter then travels downward and ventrally until it joins the bladder, which lies in a *suprapubic* position (above the symphysis pubis or pubic arch) in the anterior part of the pelvic cavity.

A diagnostic test frequently ordered for patients on urologic units is the *KUB,* and the student should realize that a KUB is an x-ray film of the urinary system: the kidneys, ureters, and bladder.

The urethra has its proximal end at the bladder neck. In the female, it is about 1½ inches long and exits distally above the vaginal opening in the perineum. In the male, it is from 8 to 10 inches long, transverses the penis, and has its external orifice at the tip of the glans penis.

RENAL CIRCULATION AND INNERVATION

The large space occupied by the liver tends to displace the right kidney downward so that it is usually a little lower than the left. Centrally located on the concave border of each kidney is a cleft called the *hilum* (see Fig. 2), which provides the avenue through which the ureter, blood vessels, and nerves enter and leave the kidney. Thus it is at the hilum that each kidney receives a large artery from the abdominal aorta—the *renal artery*—and relinquishes a large vein that empties into the inferior vena cava, the *renal vein.* In discussions of renal circulation, it is the cortical or outermost part of the kidney parenchyma that should receive initial attention. It is in the cortex that the glomeruli and convoluted tubules are located;

these structures make up the *nephrons*, which are the structural and functional units of the kidney. There are about one million nephrons in each kidney.

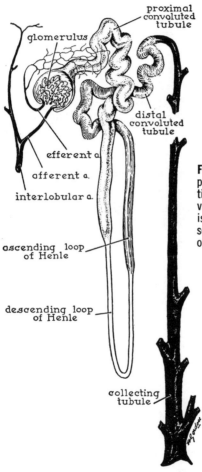

Fig. 3. The nephron. In this simplified diagram, the normal relation of the loop of Henle to the vascular pole of the glomerulus is omitted (From Ham and Leeson. Histology, 4th ed. Courtesy of J. P. Lippincott, Co.)

The nephron (see Fig. 3) begins as the glomerulus. In some references it is also referred to as either the renal corpuscle or the malpighian body. The glomerular space or Bowman's capsule forms a continuum with the lumen of the *renal tubule*—a long cylinder of tortuous configuration which is comprised of three sections: the *proximal convoluted tubule*, the *loop of Henle*, and the *distal convoluted tubule*. The distal convoluted tubule marks the end of the nephron. The collecting ducts and papillary ducts are located in the medullary part of the parenchyma and will be discussed later in the chapter.

Upon entering the hilum, the renal artery divides and subdivides into numerous branches that form minute arteries which travel to the junction between the cortex and medulla. Then these branches pass outward through the cortex where *afferent arterioles* carry blood to the glomeruli. Once an afferent arteriole has entered a glomerulus, it divides further into a dense cluster of capillaries that are interconnected by short communicating channels and surrounded by Bowman's capsule. These capillaries merge, emptying into an *efferent arteriole* which continues its travel in one of two ways: (1) the efferent arterioles of most glomeruli subdivide into networks of capillaries surrounding the convoluted tubules as they lie in the cortex; (2) the efferent arterioles of the glomeruli closest to the junction between the cortex and medulla divide into groups of capillaries which descend into the medulla and then return to the cortex (following a course similar to that of the loops of Henle). After following one of the aforementioned routes, these capillaries reunite to form cortical and medullary venous systems which converge, forming veins that will eventually merge into the *renal vein*. The renal vein exists at the hilum and empties into the inferior vena cava.

The nerve supply of the urinary system arises from many widespread sources—a phenomenon characteristic of the autonomic nervous system. Therefore, to permit easier understanding, the innervation of the kidney parenchyma, ureters, and bladder will be discussed consecutively rather than collectively.

The nerves to the kidney parenchyma arise from five sources (Mitchell, 1950) which converge to become a complex referred to as the *renal plexus* (see Fig. 4). However, this rich nerve supply seems to play a relatively minor role in the functioning of the parenchymal structures. The majority of the nerves comprising the renal plexus lie near the renal artery, but a few come into proximity with this vessel only in the hilum of the kidney. It is these nerves that accompany the renal arteries and their branches. They have some control over the circulation of the blood in the kidney by regulating the lumen of the small blood vessels. Experimentation has demonstrated that stimulation of these nerves produces a marked reduction in blood flow and, in some cases, anuria (absence or suppression of urine formation) (Winton, 1959).

Starting at the level of the kidney, the proximal segment of each ureter receives fibers from the sympathetic nervous system (from the renal plexus), while the central segment of each ureter receives fibers from the spermatic (or ovarian) plexus. The distal segment of each ureter receives fibers from the hypogastric nerves. Urine is propelled from the kidney pelvis down the ureters and into the bladder by peristaltic waves. It is the sympathetic innervation which exerts a predominantly motor effect on the ureters, although research has demonstrated that inhibitory fibers are also derived from the sympathetic nervous system. In addition to their motor effect on the ureters, the sympathetic nerves cause contraction of the ureteral orifices. Parasympathetic fibers to the ureters have not been demonstrated.

As for the innervation of the bladder (see Fig. 4), that organ receives efferent nerves from the sympathetic and parasympathetic pathways. To clarify terminology again, the external layer of the bladder musculature is referred to as the *detrusor muscle*, and the sympathetic nervous system furnishes the detrusor muscle with *inhibitory fibers*. The trigone, internal

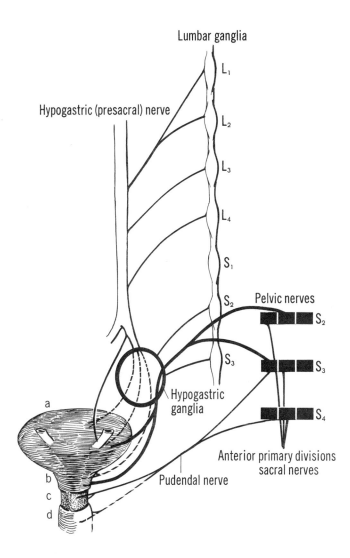

Fig. 4. The renal plexus and the innervation of the bladder. a. The bladder. b. The internal sphincter. c. The posterior urethra. d. The external sphincter.

sphincter, and smooth muscle of the proximal part of the urethra are provided with *motor fibers* which also come from the sympathetic pathway. (Learmonth, 1931). Parasympathetic nerves exert a reciprocal action by supplying *motor fibers* to the detrusor muscle to govern its tone and contractibility, and *inhibitory fibers* to the internal sphincter.

The external sphincter is innervated through the pudendal nerves. The pelvic nerves contain the afferent fibers that play an important role in the reflex movements of the bladder; the pudendal nerves contain those for the movements of the urethra. The hypogastric nerves contain *no afferent pathways* for any of the essential reflex actions. However, the feeling of pain travels mainly in the hypogastrics. The feeling of discomfort from bladder distention is conveyed by the pelvic *and* hypogastric nerves.

When *cystometrics* are done—the procedure by which the bladder is filled with solution to estimate its capacity and pressure reaction—the sensation of pressure or filling is carried mainly by the pelvic nerves. When "hot and cold" cystometrics are done, the bladder is first filled with a solution at room temperature and then with a solution that has been chilled. The thermal sensations are also carried in the pelvic nerves.

THE FORMATION OF URINE

Maintenance of a normal arterial pressure range is important in insuring adequate blood flow through the kidneys; concern about adequate blood flow through the kidneys is justifiable because the process of urine formation begins with filtration of the plasma in the glomerulus. Actually, urine formation is characterized by three distinct processes: *glomerular filtration*, *tubular reabsorption*, and *tubular secretion*. These processes will be discussed consecutively.

Blood carried by the renal arteries and its branches is

filtered in the glomeruli. The amounts of water and solutes filtered are dependent upon these substances' concentration in the plasma *and* the rate of glomerular filtration. The glomerular filtration rate (GFR) is determined by the pressure in the glomerular capillaries and *not* by the blood or plasma flow. This must be emphasized because a review of the literature may lead to confusion. It has been demonstrated that constriction of the afferent arterioles decreases the GFR by decreasing flow and pressure in the glomerulus, whereas dilatation increases both. However, it has also been observed that the behavior of the efferent arteriole is independent of the afferent. The lumen of efferent arterioles is about half the size of the afferent; when they are constricted, blood flow is diminished but the filtration pressure is increased. On the other hand, dilatation of the efferent arterioles causes an increase in the blood flow but decreases the filtration pressure. The renal nerves influence the regulation of arteriolar behavior and thus help to maintain a stable GFR, but they are not essential to this stability. The kidney seems to be able to make spontaneous adjustments within its arterioles, and this intrinsic ability —independent of outside control—is called *autoregulation* (Winton, 1959).

Glomerular capillaries are distinguishable from those of other capillary networks because (1) they are dispersed between two arterioles (an afferent and an efferent), (2) they maintain a high hydrostatic pressure, and (3) they have high permeability. The filtrate separated from the blood flowing through the glomerular capillaries is considered protein-free, but it does contain those crystalloid components of the plasma that are capable of passing through a semipermeable membrane. These substances include electrolytes—such as sodium, chlorides, water, potassium, bicarbonate, phosphate, calcium, and ammonia—as well as nonelectrolytes such as urea, creatinine, uric acid, and glucose (White et al., 1959). Actually, traces of protein may enter the filtrate because of the normal imperfections in the capillary endothelium, but they are usually completely removed during the process of absorption so that no protein is found in the urine. The filtrate is conveyed from the glomerular capillaries into the space of Bowman's capsule. The capsule acts as a portal of entry into the lumen of the proximal tubule, and the net filtration pressure forces the filtrate through the tubule—where it is greatly modified in volume and composition through the processes of reabsorption and secretion. Of the 125 ml or more of glomerular filtrate formed per minute, approximately 15 ml reaches the distal tubule. Another interesting fact to note here is that the filtrate has a pH of about 7.4 and a specific gravity of about 1.010—values close to the usual range seen in the finished product, urine.

Quantitatively speaking, the most crucial process executed by the kidney is the reabsorption of sodium salts and water. Most of the glomerular filtrate is reabsorbed in the proximal tubule, and the active process by which sodium ions are absorbed is the highlight of this process. It is believed that the movement of chlorides is secondary to the transport of sodium. The movement of water from the tubule lumen, unlike that of sodium, is believed to be a passive process resulting from osmotic dictates initiated by the removal of salt; water will diffuse through the highly permeable tubular lining so that the fluid within the lumen maintains the same osmotic pressure as the peritubular tissue and blood. Thus the process of tubular reabsorption can be divided into two categories: passive and active reabsorption. And the most significant accomplishment of the proximal tubule is the return to the circulating blood of the previously filtered water and solutes necessary for metabolism (Lamdin, 1959).

The movement of any substance across a semipermeable membrane is considered passive when no energy is expended by the cells to effect that movement. The passive process taking place in the proximal tubule is most comprehensively explained by the *gradients of concentration theory*. In essence, this theory refers to solute concentration differences between the filtrate within the proximal tubule and its surrounding environment: the interstitial fluid and plasma. The reabsorption of urea is typical of such a passive process; it can be explained entirely by gradients of concentration. A schematic diagram (see Fig. 5) has been provided to make the concept clearer.

During the course of water transport out of the tubular lumen, when there develops a greater concentration of solute (in this case urea) *within the lumen* than the concentration of that solute in the surrounding environment, a *concentration gradient* is created. If the tubular endothelium is permeable to the solute in question, the solute will diffuse from the lumen out into the interstitial fluid and blood; *the solute passes from an area of higher concentration to an area of lower concentration.*

The processes which require the expenditure of energy for the movement of certain solutes and which cannot be explained by the gradients of concentration mechanism are termed *active reabsorption* processes. The movement of glucose, phosphate, sulfate, and uric acid is typical of this activity as transport of these substances is accomplished *against* a concentration gradient—with solutes passing from areas of lower concentration *to* areas of higher concentration. In other words, the cells must work to accomplish the reabsorption of these solutes. The net result of both passive and active reabsorptive processes in the proximal tubule is a modification of the glomerular filtrate making it isotonic with the blood (Mostofi and Smith, 1966).

As the isotonic filtrate leaves the proximal portion of the convoluted tubule to enter the first segment or descending portion of the loop of Henle, the cells of this *thin limb* of the loop are quite permeable to water. This, then, is an area of *high*

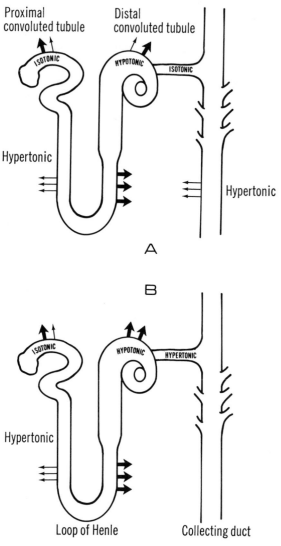

Fig. 5. Diagrammatic representation of the areas of active reabsorption of sodium chloride and the passive movement of water. Heavy arrows indicate the movement of sodium chloride and the thin arrows indicate the movement of water. The concentration of sodium salts around the loops is high; therefore, the passive outward movement of water from the thin limb of the loop represents an attempt to reestablish osmotic equilibrium. Note the changes in tonicity as the filtrate travels through the tubule. A. The indicated changes in tonicity yield concentrated urine. B. The indicated changes in tonicity yield dilute urine.

water permeability, and water diffuses out (is reabsorbed) making the filtrate *hypertonic*. This outward migration of water is influenced by the activity taking place in the ascending limb: the active reabsorption of sodium in an area of *low water permeability*. Part of the loops with their surrounding blood vessels (the vasa recta) and supporting tissue are located in the renal medulla. These portions provide a system for conveying salt to the interstitial tissue of that area. The tubular cells there are also less permeable to water, and the loops must accomplish their task by actively transporting sodium (and chlorides) in an area of low water permeability. Further on along the ascending limb, more sodium is transported out into the peritubular region.

When the process of reabsorption of sodium to cortical and medullary areas is conceptualized, and the relatively long segment of low water permeability along the loops is considered, it seems inevitable that the thin limb of the loops would relinquish water to this hypertonic environment in an attempt to reestablish osmotic equilibrium. Further, if the filtrate leaving the descending limb has been made *hypertonic* from the loss of water, then that same filtrate—losing sodium but little water in the medulla, and giving up more sodium and solute but little water as it reenters the cortex in the ascending limb—is made *hypotonic* by the time it reaches the distal convoluted tubule (see Fig. 5). Micropuncture technique has confirmed this (Gottschalk and Mylle, 1959).

It may be wise at this juncture to refer to Figure 3 for a graphic illustration of the proximity of the ascending and descending limbs of the loop of Henle. It should also be remembered that the concentration of sodium salts around the loops is high, and this accounts for the reabsorption of water from the thin limb. The *passive* movement of water from the loop in an area of high water permeability is a consequence of the *active* transport of sodium salt.

TUBULAR SECRETION AND THE INFLUENCE OF ADH

Tubular secretion is the term given to the processes by which solutes are removed from the peritubular fluid and returned to the lumen of the tubule. It would seem that the activities of the proximal tubules and loops of Henle are predominantly unselective in character, being governed for the most part by the principles of osmosis. Thus the task of the distal convoluted tubules and the collecting ducts is that of determining the ultimate concentration of the urine. The *specific gravity* is used as the index of urine concentration and dilution, and a value of 1.008 to 1.010 is approximately isotonic with plasma. Thus the specific gravity is often of aid to the physician in determining the condition and/or treatment of an individual patient.

The distal convoluted tubules also reabsorb water; in addition to water they reabsorb sodium, chlorides, potassium, phosphates, endogenous creatinine, and urea—returning them to the peritubular capillaries, to be retained in the body. The remaining solutes and water in the peritubular fluid which are not needed by the body are secreted (returned) into the lumen of the tubules to be excreted in urine. Then the urine leaves the distal convoluted tubules and enters the collecting tubules.

The discriminatory function within the distal tubule which determines urinary concentration is influenced greatly by a hormone produced in the hypothalamus and stored in the posterior part of the pituitary gland—the antidiuretic hormone (ADH). The processes which are concerned with the reabsorption of water within the proximal and distal tubules possess one basic similarity and one basic difference. Their activities are similar in that the passive reabsorption of water follows the active reabsorption of sodium, leading to a reduction of the volume of the original filtrate. However, a significant difference is the influence of ADH. Water reabsorption in the proximal convoluted tubule is completely independent of ADH: a water-permeable membrane accomplishes its movement. However, the porous walls of the distal convoluted tubule open for the diffusion of water under the influence of ADH. It is a water-impermeable membrane that is present in the distal tubule, and ADH is essential for the alteration of permeability to permit the movement of water. With the amount of water reabsorbed being monitored by the action of ADH on the porous epithelium of the distal convoluted tubule, the filtrate may be further reduced in volume but isotonicity is maintained.

As for the mechanism of the action of ADH, it is believed that the solute-water ratio (which can change the osmotic pressure) of body fluids affects certain receptor cells in the hypothalamus, leading to the transmission of nervous impulses to the pituitary gland. These nervous impulses influence the release of ADH from the posterior part of the gland. Thus a rise in the solute concentration of body fluids—as a consequence of water loss or solute gain—results in an increase of osmotic pressure which is perceived by the receptor cells in the hypothalamus. These in turn stimulate ADH secretion and the ADH is carried by the blood to the kidneys—resulting in increased water permeability of the distal tubular walls. Water is thereby allowed to move out of the tubule into the interstitium, and this movement results in the manufacture of concentrated urine. This means that the bulk of the water filtered from the blood has been reabsorbed for use by the body, and body fluid is restored to normal. The mechanism of ADH secretion usually works as described. However, under abnormal conditions (such as the experience of fear and nausea, or trauma), or under the influence of certain drugs, ADH may be secreted regardless of the osmotic pressure of the body fluids.

Following the course of the tubular filtrate which leaves the distal convoluted tubule, it enters the collecting ducts which traverse the medulla. Here additional amounts of water are reabsorbed and returned to the peritubular area, and this is considered to be the last stage in the formation of urine. This area acts to accomplish a further concentration of the urine, but this function is also dependent on the influence of ADH. (In addition to ADH, the parathyroid hormone may have an effect on the regulation of renal function, but this will be discussed in detail in the chapter on calculi and calculus formation).

In addition to the specific gravity of urine, the pH is often referred to. The normal breakdown of foods ingested is a source of acid for the human body. The normal balanced diet provides more acid than alkaline potential, and kidney action in maintaining the acid-base balance of the body is accomplished by the regulation of the amount of acid or alkali excreted in urine. The symbol pH indicates the hydrogen ion concentration of a solution, the value of which determines the acidity of that solution. A pH of 7 tells us that there is neutrality, and the solution is neither acid nor alkaline in character. It is important for the student to remember that the *lower* the numerical value, the *more acid* the solution and the *higher* the numerical value of the pH, the *more alkaline* the solution. Thus a pH of 4 denotes a higher acid value than a pH of 6, whereas a pH of 10 denotes a higher alkaline value than a pH of 8. The normal pH of urine is below 7, and it is *the reabsorption of bicarbonate from the glomerular filtrate which determines the pH of the urine.* When the urine is free of bicarbonate it is acid and will have a pH lower than 7, but when bicarbonate remains in the filtrate—when tubular capacity to reabsorb hydrogen ion is impaired—the urine is alkaline (is seen to have a value higher than 7).

After the urine leaves the collecting ducts, it flows to the papillary ducts of the pyramids which empty into the calyces. From here, the urine enters the pelvis of the kidney and *peristaltic waves* convey the urine down the ureters to the bladder, which serves as a reservoir. The calyces, pelvis, ureters, bladder, and urethra are considered to be the *collecting system* of the kidneys and are not to be confused with the structures comprising the parenchymal (actively functioning) system.

THE PROCESS OF MICTURITION

Strong contractions of the bladder musculature with concurrent relaxation of the internal sphincter that is followed by the opening of the external sphincter are the integrated processes which permit voiding. The bladder has a capacity of from 300 to 500 ml, the capacity being dependent on the tone of the detrusor muscle and on its reflex excitability.

When 200 to 350 ml of urine has accumulated, tension on the walls of the bladder from the increased internal pressure *(intravesical pressure)* provides the stimulus for the detrusor to contract. The *pelvic nerves* serve as the pathway for this reflex; the center is located in the hindbrain. As the detrusor contracts, the internal sphincter relaxes. Urine coursing through the urethra sets up the stimulus that sustains the contraction of the detrusor until intravesical pressure has decreased. The *pudendal (pudic) nerves* transport the afferent limb of this reflex to the hindbrain and from the hindbrain the efferent limb is carried by way of the pelvic nerves. In other words, as long as urine continues to flow through the urethra as the result of the bladder's initial contraction, that first reflex (initiated by the pelvic nerves) will be maintained by a second reflex (initiated by the pudendal nerves) until the bladder has emptied its contents.

The urine coursing through the urethra sets up a stimulus which initiates still another reflex which brings about the relaxation of the external sphincter. The center for this reflex, however, is in the sacral part of the spinal cord and not in the hindbrain. Both afferent and efferent limbs of this reflex are carried by the pudendal nerves. Relaxation of the external sphincter is also influenced by nerve impulses conveyed via the pelvic nerves when the intravesical pressure increases. Again, the spinal cord is the center for this reflex, and the pudendal nerves transport the efferent limb of the reflex.

Though it would seem that micturition is completely reflex in nature, it is normally initiated or terminated at will. Control by the higher nervous centers—in the hypothalamus and cerebral cortex—accounts for this fact. The role played by the abdominal muscles should also be considered at this time. An increase of pressure within the abdominal cavity (such as may be caused by coughing, sneezing, or the act of defecation) may force the escape of urine from the bladder into the urethra. This in turn serves as enough of a stimulus to start micturition, and will power must be employed to prevent it. Micturition is completely reflex in nature only when trauma or disease severs the bladder's connection to the cortical centers of the brain.

REFERENCES

1. Best, C. H., and Taylor, N. B. The Physiological Basis of Medical Practice, 7th ed. Baltimore, The Williams & Wilkins Co., 1961.
2. Boyarsky, S., et. al. Does the ureter have nervous control? J. Urol., 97:627–632, 1967.
3. Creevy, C. D. An Outline of Urology. Minneapolis, Burgess Publishing Co., 1963.
4. Gottschalk, C. W., and Mylle, M. Micropuncture study of the mammalian urinary concentrating mechanism: Evidence for the countercurrent hypothesis. Amer. J. Physiol., 196:927, 1959.

5. Holmes, G. Introduction to Clinical Neurology. Baltimore, The Williams & Wilkins Co., 1947, pp. 157–160.
6. Lamdin, E. Mechanisms of urinary concentration and dilution. Arch. Intern. Med. (Chicago), 103:644–668, 1959.
7. Learmonth, J. R. A contribution to the neurophysiology of the urinary bladder in man. Brain, 54:147–175, 1931.
8. Mitchell, G. A. G. The nerve supply of the kidneys. Acta Anat., 10:1–32, 1950.
9. Mostofi, F. K., and Smith, D. E., eds. The Kidney. Baltimore, The Williams & Wilkins Co., 1966.
10. White, A., Handler, P., Smith, E., and Stetten, D. Principles of Biochemistry, 2nd ed. New York, McGraw-Hill Book Company, 1959.
11. Winton, F. R. Present concepts of the renal circulation. Arch. Intern. Med. (Chicago), 103:495–501, 1959.

3

Urologic Equipment

Every specialty in medicine has equipment especially adapted for its use, and urology is no exception. Instrumentation of the urinary tract is often indicated, and, as intubation (insertion of a tube or catheter) should be anticipated, this chapter will present a discussion of the equipment most frequently used in the clinical situation, as well as the concurrent and subsequent implications for nursing care.

During the course of nursing education, the student will undoubtedly observe catheters being used. These catheters come in different sizes, and the sizes are usually designated by a numeral which is followed by the letters *Fr* (for example, 18 Fr, 16 Fr, 26 Fr, etc.). The Fr stands for *French*, a unit of measure: one French unit being equal to one-third of a millimeter. This French unit refers to the *diameter of the outside of the catheter.* The student would do well to remember that the female urethra will accommodate a larger catheter than the male urethra. It should also be noted that catheters are named to describe their appearance, and that they vary in shape as well as in size. They may be straight, curved, or angulated to meet the needs of the urologist. The holes appearing in them are called *eyes*.

CATHETERS

A catheter which is able to hold itself in a cavity independent of external supportive agents is referred to as a *self-retaining catheter* (see Fig. 1a). The most commonly used—and possibly most familiar—self-retaining catheter is the Foley catheter. It is most frequently used as a urethral catheter (inserted to drain the bladder), but it may be used postoperatively as a cystostomy tube (inserted directly into the bladder through a suprapubic incision) or as a nephrostomy tube (inserted directly into the kidney pelvis through a lumbar incision). The Foley catheter is usually straight and of latex rubber with a smooth, rounded tip. It has a balloon near the tip which can be inflated (through a channel at the end, opposite the tip) by the introduction of air, sterile water, or sterile sodium chloride solution; and it may have one or more eyes. Foley catheters come in various sizes, may be angulated, and may have a balloon (or bag) with a capacity of 5 ml or more. When inflated, the 5-ml bag is ordinarily large enough to retain the Foley catheter in the bladder; the bags which have a capacity of 30 ml or more are usually inserted when hemostasis at the bladder neck or in the prostatic fossa is desired.

Most hospitals have a preferred procedure for the catheterization of patients and for the insertion of Foley catheters. When the student is in the clinical situation, therefore, the procedure manual should be used as reference for a detailed description of the treatment; this usually includes the name of the solution to be utilized for cleansing, as well as the preferred method of insertion.

Once the Foley catheter has been inserted, the nurse should secure it to the inner aspect of either thigh with ad-

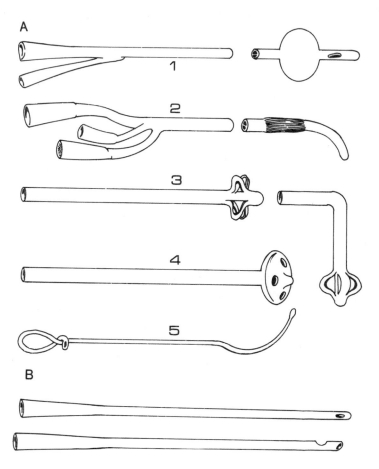

Fig. 1A. Self-retaining catheters. 1. The Foley catheter. 2. The three-way Foley catheter. 3. The Malecot catheter. 4. The Pezzer catheter. These catheters are able to maintain themselves in cavities. They come in various sizes and may be straight or angulated. Both types of Foley catheters are introduced into a cavity and the self-retaining balloon is inflated thereafter. The self-retaining protuberance at the tip of the Malecot and Pezzer must be elongated with a stylet (5) which is passed through the lumen before insertion. After insertion, the stylet is removed and the protuberance secures the catheter in place. **1B.** Straight catheters. The straight catheter may have a single eye or many eyes; it may have a round tip or a whistle tip. These catheters are not self-retaining and must be secured with adhesive tape when being utilized as indwelling tubes.

hesive (or Scotch) tape or—for the male patient—to the fly of the pajama pants. Through these steps, the possibility of tension on the Foley catheter is minimized. If the inner aspect of the thigh is to be used, the nurse should ask the patient to externally rotate the thigh *before* the catheter is taped to it (see Fig. 2a). In this way, when the patient is ambulatory, the movement of the legs will not result in a pulling of the catheter. Many patients perspire in the thigh region and such moisture often prevents adhesive from sticking to the skin in that area. This can be quite discouraging to the conscientious student who is trying to prevent dislodgement of the catheter. Application of a *small* amount of tincture of benzoin to the desired area prior to positioning of the tape will enhance the adhesive potential. If securing the catheter to the pajama pants fly is more feasible, a small piece of half-inch tape may be placed around the proximal portion of the Foley at the bifurcation (i.e., the area of branching of the balloon-inflating channel and drainage lumen), which forms a tab that can be secured with a pin (see Fig. 2b).

When it is time for a Foley catheter to be removed, the self-retaining balloon must be deflated. This is accomplished by removal of the solution or air retained in it. The nurse may withdraw the catheter from a male patient by giving firm support to the glans with one gloved hand while gently—but quickly—pulling the catheter out with the other hand (see Fig. 3). Such removal when ordered may be accomplished with a minimum of discomfort if—immediately before the catheter is to be pulled out—the patient is instructed to take a slow deep breath. Then, as the patient exhales, the nurse pulls the catheter out. The deep breathing serves to assist the patient in relaxing. It also serves as the distraction which aids in making this treatment less traumatic. The patient's attention is momentarily diverted to the deep breathing and he is thus less aware of the pull of the catheter as it is being removed. The same technique may be utilized when a Foley

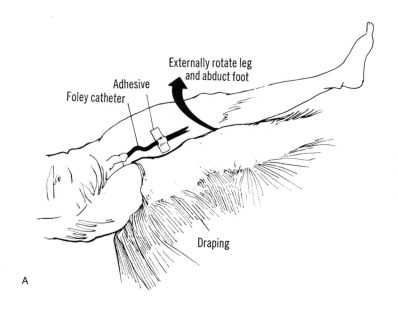

Externally rotate leg
and abduct foot

Adhesive
Foley catheter

Draping

A

Fig. 2A. Method by which a catheter may be secured to the thigh. The thigh should be externally rotated **before** the catheter is taped to it. The portion of the thigh which will accommodate the tape should be shaved if necessary.

catheter is to be removed from a female patient, the gloved hand affording gentle support to the labia surrounding the urinary meatus.

Three-way Foley catheters are utilized when irrigation as well as drainage of the bladder is desired. This Foley is so named because of the three arms that branch from the end opposite the tip. One arm is connected to the channel which inflates the bag; another may be connected to the prescribed drainage system; and the third arm may be connected to an irrigating system to allow fluid and/or medication to be instilled into the bladder. Three-way Foleys also come in various sizes graduated on the French scale.

B

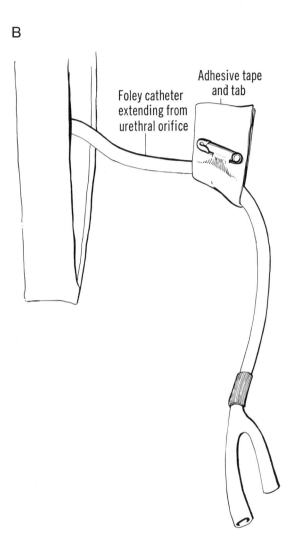

Foley catheter
extending from
urethral orifice

Adhesive tape
and tab

Fig. 2B. Method by which a catheter may be secured to the fly of pajama pants. Note that when the adhesive tape secured to the catheter is allowed to form a tab, a pin can easily be inserted into the tab and then onto the **fly** of the pajama pants.

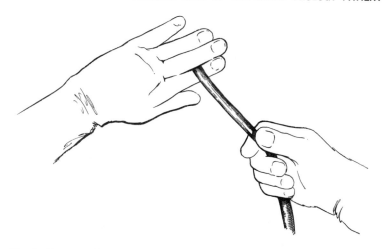

Fig. 3. Removal of a catheter from the urethra. Note the position of the hand being used to support the area surrounding the tube while it is being removed. Support should also be afforded when a nephrostomy or cystostomy tube is being removed.

Another self-retaining catheter is the Pezzer or mushroom catheter. This latex catheter with the mushroom shaped bulb comprising the tip is most commonly used as a nephrostomy or cystostomy tube. However, it may be used as an indwelling urethral catheter in female patients when gross hematuria and clots are present. The Pezzer catheter usually has two or more eyes in the mushroom, and is inserted with a stylet—that is, a metal probe that is used to stiffen a catheter to facilitate its passage (see Fig. 1a). When the stylet is introduced within the lumen of the Pezzer, the mushroom tip can be elongated and passage of the catheter is facilitated. After the catheter has entered the desired cavity, removal of the stylet returns the rim of the mushroom to its natural shape and the catheter is thereby held in place. When the Pezzer catheter is to be removed, the patient is usually instructed to take a deep breath and—while the surrounding area is being supported with one hand—the catheter is pulled out gently but quickly with the other hand as the patient exhales. Internal tissues are seldom traumatized by removal in this manner because the catheter is made of a soft and pliable synthetic rubber. Pezzer catheters come in various sizes (10 Fr to 40 Fr) and may be straight or angulated.

The Malecot catheter (see Fig. 1a) is also made of latex and has a tip comprised of two or more winglike projections which serve to hold it in position. It is also frequently used as a nephrostomy or cystostomy tube, and is inserted and removed in the same manner as the Pezzer.

In addition to catheters with a self-retaining protuberance near or for the tip, catheters without self-retaining properties are utilized on urologic units. Straight catheters (see Fig. 1b) with rounded tips fall under this category. They may be single or many eyed and may be used to catheterize the bladder or to facilitate the drainage of a cutaneous ureterostomy.* Straight catheters with *whistle tips* (see Fig. 1b) may also be used to drain a ureter after renal surgery, but they are particularly suitable when hematuria and clots are noted because a whistle tip is wider than the size of the regular catheter eye—thereby providing better drainage when blocking of the tube by clots is anticipated. These catheters are usually secured with tape when they are to be utilized as indwelling tubes.

Angulated catheters with whistle tips often serve as cystostomy tubes. They are inserted into the bladder after the suprapubic incision has been made and are held in place by a suture. These tubes come in sizes up to 40 Fr.

The coudé tip is a curved tip which may be either smooth or elliptical (see Fig. 1a). Straight catheters with coudé tips are used primarily for catheterization of female patients—the smooth, curved tip making them easier to pass. The curved elliptical tip is used only when the doctor encounters diffi-

---

* After a ureter has been surgically separated from the bladder, the formation of a *ureteral* opening on the abdominal wall is referred to as a cutaneous ureterostomy. (The *ureter* should not be confused with the *urethra*.) Indications for such a procedure will be discussed later.

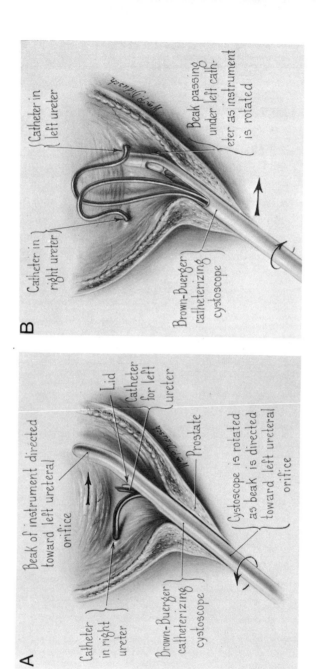

Fig. 4A, B, C, D. Cystoscopy. Note the ureteral catheters being threaded up into the ureters. (Courtesy of the American Cystoscopy Makers, Inc., Pelham Manor, N.Y.)

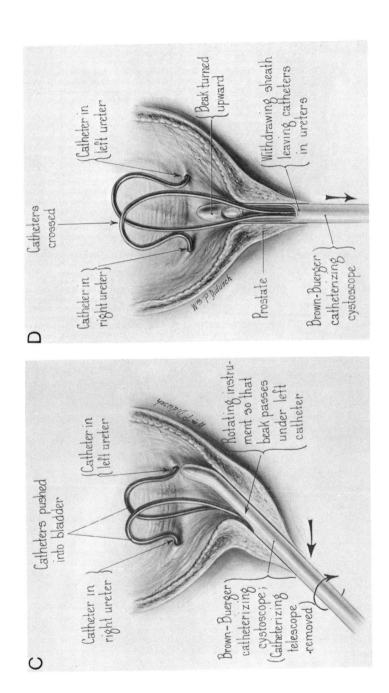

C

Catheters pushed into bladder

Catheter in left ureter

Catheter in right ureter

Rotating instrument so that beak passes under left catheter

Wm. P. Didusch

Brown-Buerger catheterizing cystoscope; (catheterizing telescope removed)

D

Catheters crossed

Catheter in left ureter

Beak turned upward

Withdrawing sheath leaving catheters in ureters

Catheter in right ureter

Wm. P. Didusch

Prostate

Brown-Buerger catheterizing cystoscope

culty in passing a catheter urethrally. The slight dilatation which occurs as the firm bulbous tip is introduced often leads to easier passage of the remaining portion of the catheter.

Ureteral catheters are obtainable in sizes 3 Fr to 12 Fr and, therefore, have the narrowest lumen of any catheter that the student will encounter on a urologic unit. The size of these catheters is compatible with the size of the lumen of the normal ureter. In addition to being narrower than other catheters, ureteral catheters are longer because they must be threaded through the urethra, past the bladder neck, and up into the ureter to the kidney pelvis. These catheters have rounded tips and many eyes; are usually firm and made of woven nylon or polyethylene substance; are radiopaque; and are calibrated to assist the doctor in determining how far it has been inserted into the ureter. Ureteral catheters are frequently utilized during cystoscopy (i.e., direct visualization of the bladder) and are passed through the working lens of the cystoscope, which is the instrument (see Fig. 4) used to accomplish this visualization. This treatment allows for catheterization of the ureter or kidney pelvis.

DILATORS

Dilators are unique in that they have no *lumen;* theirs is primarily a stretching function, not a draining function. They come in sets that contain instruments ranging in sizes from 8 Fr through 30 Fr. Dilation is accomplished by a technique of graduated insertion and withdrawal of instruments, beginning with the narrowest dilator in the set and ending with the widest. Dilators are most frequently ordered for urologic patients when there is stricture (narrowing) of the urethra —the stricture being either congenital or secondary to a disease process. Occasionally, ureteral dilatation may be indicated because of ureteral stricture.

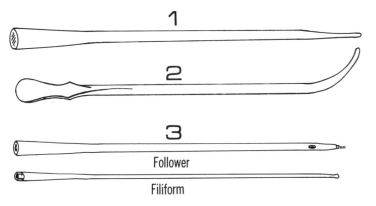

Fig. 5. Dilators: 1. The Bougie. 2. The Sound. 3. The Philips. Dilators have no lumen because their primary function is to stretch a lumen, not to drain a cavity. With the Philips dilator, it is the filiform which accomplishes the initial dilation of the urethra.

There are basically three types of dilators: the sound, the bougie, and the Philips dilator (see Fig. 5). Of the three dilators mentioned, the nurse will most frequently encounter the *sound*. A sound has the contour of a latex catheter whose distal portion is curved, but since it has *no lumen* and is made of *metal*, it is inflexible. It is understandable then for the doctor to order an analgesic to be administered prior to a dilation treatment. When such premedication is ordered, the nurse should remember to pull up the side rails on the bed after the patient has received the medication (the same safety precautions instituted for the preoperative patient). This is specifically applicable for patients in the older age group. When facilities permit, it is also advisable for the nurse to prepare the set-up in the treatment room rather than at the bedside— especially if the patient is in a semiprivate or ward room. Some patients find the treatment painful and outcries from such patients are upsetting to the other individuals sharing the room. It should be remembered that dilation of the urethra may be quite uncomfortable and often *painful* for the male patient, and the apprehension manifested by most patients prior to the treatment seems to compound the discomfort.

Bougies are impregnated, woven dilators which are more flexible than sounds. Their passage imposes some discomfort, but is usually not so painful for the patient. Like sounds, they also come in sets.

The *filiform* and *follower* comprise the two parts of the Philips dilator. The filiform is of very fine and flexible material and looks like a thin probe. It may be from 6 to 9 inches in length, and it terminates in a base into which the follower screws. The filiform is usually indicated when severe urethral strictures are encountered in male patients. In this circumstance, a dilator smaller than 8 Fr is required if the constricted area is to be bypassed; the filiform is invaluable because it is usually obtainable in sizes 1 Fr to 6 Fr. The follower may also be a dilator larger in size than the filiform preceding it, its passage expediting the desired stretching procedure. However, most often followers have a lumen and one eye near the tip that screws into the filiform. These followers are also larger in size than the filiforms which precede them—usually ranging from 12 Fr to 24 Fr—and are of great importance in relieving the symptoms of acute urinary retention when a severe stricture causes obstruction to the outflow of urine. The filiform is passed transurethrally (dilating the passageway through the stricture) into the bladder; the adherent follower with eye and lumen enter thereafter. When the follower is attached to a drainage system, the distended bladder may be emptied. Since the follower is not a self-retaining catheter, it must be taped into place to remain securely in the bladder cavity. Often part of a strip of tape will be placed so that the tip of the follower that protrudes from the glans is encircled; then the entire penile shaft is encircled with the remainder of the adhesive strip so that the follower may be held in place. Care is always taken to insure that the tape encircling the penis is loose enough to avoid gangrene.

Mucoid exudate from the walls of the urethra may ooze from the urethral orifice encircling the follower. This exudate —representing tissue reaction secondary to intubation—may collect around the tip of the glans and adhere to the tape. The maintenance of good hygiene is thus made a difficult task, but secondary infection is not common because the Philips dilator is seldom left in place longer than 72 hours. Once the acute symptoms are resolved, the patient is usually "sounded" (dilated with sounds) and a self-retaining catheter—a Foley—is inserted. Should the exudate become a problem, a solution of 60 ml peroxide, 30 ml surgical soap, and 30 ml water may be poured over the area and gently wiped off with a sponge. Cleansing may thus be effected with little danger of dislodgment of the tape or irritation of the glans. Often the patient can be taught to do this and the student need only provide the solution and sponges for his use. Directions for cleansing should be given concisely, and terminology should be simple. A statement such as "You may wash off the colored discharge from around the tube by pouring the solution over the area where the tube comes out of you" will be explicit enough to prevent embarrassment to both patient and student. However, the patient must be cautioned against wetting the entire penile shaft since this will cause the tape to slip off, thereby dislodging the follower.

DRAINAGE AND IRRIGATING SYSTEMS

In addition to the equipment that the nurse will encounter, there are procedures and treatments which are of prime importance in the management of the patient on a urologic service. Obstruction is the term used to describe blockage of the free flow of urine through the ureter, bladder, and urethra. Such blockage is usually secondary to stricture, tumor, or calculus formation. When the normal physiologic drainage system of the kidney is obstructed, the patient is predisposed to impaired renal function resulting from infection secondary to stasis (e.g., cystitis or pyelonephritis) or from increased pressure on the kidney parenchymal substance (i.e., hydronephrosis). The patient is also subjected to the discomfort and/or pain inherent in obstruction. When obstruction occurs in the lower urinary tract—in the urethra or at the bladder neck—the patient experiences the suprapubic discomfort of retention. If the obstruction occurs at the UP junction (ureteropelvic junction, where the ureter meets the kidney pelvis), within the ureter, or at the UV junction (ureterovesical junction, where the ureter enters the bladder), the patient experiences flank pain.

To prevent these complications or to reverse their course if they are already present, an *artificial drainage system* must be provided through intubation of the urinary tract—bypassing the obstruction. Often after the cavity has been successfully intubated, the doctor may want to cleanse that cavity or to administer medication topically (i.e., directly to the site). An *irrigating system* must be provided to accomplish this. Irrigating systems make it possible for the urinary tract to be cleansed of potentially harmful sediment and may also serve as an invaluable adjunctive vehicle through which inflammatory processes of the urinary tract may be treated. The ensuing discussion is applicable to any catheter dwelling within the urinary tract, regardless of the cavity it drains.

An indwelling urethral catheter is usually connected to a urinary drainage system; of the several drainage set-ups available to the doctor, the choice made in any given situation is dependent upon the needs of the patient. Although drainage systems may differ, the nurse should remember that air must be allowed to enter and escape the apparatus if a closed cavity is to be drained without the aid of suction. Stagnation occurs when urine in the cavity being drained does not displace the air in the tubing or in the drainage receptacle, and this stagnation or stasis will predispose the patient to infection.

The set-up most commonly utilized in urology is the *gravity drainage system*. The purpose of the gravity drainage system is to evacuate a closed cavity through a strategic utilization of the pull of gravity. One end of the drainage tubing should be connected to the indwelling catheter and the other allowed to drain directly into a collecting receptacle. When the tubing is allowed to sag below the level of the collecting receptacle (see Fig. 6), the upward turn of the tubing as it enters the receptacle creates an *antigravity* system. This defeats the purpose of the set-up and predisposes the patient to stasis. There are two types of gravity drainage systems: the *straight gravity drainage system* and the *vented gravity drainage system*. With the straight gravity drainage system, the indwelling catheter is attached to a length of tubing which runs directly into a collecting receptacle. The collecting receptacle is vented in some way to allow for the displacement of air from the system. The main function of this system is to provide maximum emptying of the intubated cavity. The drainage tubing is usually quite long and, therefore, may hang below the level of the lip of the collecting receptacle or coil (loop) on itself after leaving bed level. To insure against this, the tubing should be looped or coiled *on the bed* and secured by a tape-tab with a pin (or a spring clip) so that when it leaves bed level it follows a straight course into the collecting receptacle (see Fig. 6). Whichever securing device is used, the drainage tubing should be fastened to the bed near the distal-most part of its coiled length so that the patient has room enough to move about and so that the tubing runs straight into the collecting receptacle. Nurses are frequently faced with the problem of maintaining this system when the patient is ambulatory. In this event, teaching the patient is always the most efficient way of dealing with the problem.

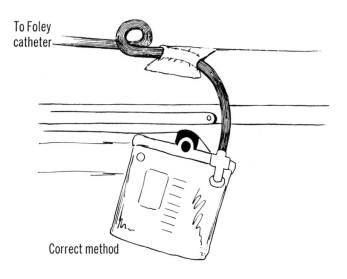

To Foley
catheter—

Correct method

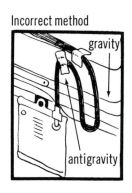

Incorrect method

gravity

antigravity

Fig. 6. The Gravity drainage system—correct and incorrect set-ups. Note that when the drainage tubing is improperly maintained, the upward flow of urine in the tubing prior to entering the collecting receptacle creates an **antigravity** system. The purpose of the set-up is thereby defeated and the patient is predisposed to stasis and infection.

The principle that should be impressed upon the patient in this teaching situation is that the urinary collecting receptacle should *always* be held (or positioned) *below* the level of the bladder. As previously described, the tape-tab applied to the tubing will permit it to be secured to the pajama pants fly, or to the leg or the hem of the nightshirt. Thus, whether the patient is walking or in a sitting position, this precaution will prevent the tubing from trailing on the floor. The coils may be supported on the lap or suspended by a rubber band which is pinned to the pajamas. If the patient is out of bed in a wheel chair, gauze slings may be suspended from the arms of the chair so that the drainage collecting receptacle will hang under the seat *lower* than bladder level and yet not obstruct the wheels.

When an indwelling catheter remains in the bladder for a period of time and is connected to a straight gravity drainage system, bladder tone and capacity are often diminished after the removal of the catheter as a result of the maximum emptying effect of the straight gravity set-up. However, this occurrence is reversible, and bladder tone and capacity return within a short time.

Because of the unique placement of an air vent, the *vented gravity drainage system* allows for a slightly slower emptying of the bladder than does the straight gravity system. In the vented gravity set-up, a glass Y connecting tube interrupts the rubber tubing approximately 6 to 8 inches from the distal end which enters the collecting receptacle; the drainage tubing enters a *closed* collecting receptacle. Thus, when the air in the collecting receptacle is displaced by urine, it travels up the same length of tubing through which urine is descending, and it escapes through the open arm of the Y connecting tube vent. The criteria of air displacement of outflow peculiar to all drainage systems is thereby met, and the functional objective of this modified gravity drainage system is realized.

To maintain this system, the nurse must not allow the glass Y connecting tube vent to hang below the level of the top of the collecting receptacle. If this is permitted, urine—instead of displaced air—will flow out the open arm of the Y connector and the system will, of course, not work. It should also be remembered that only a *closed* collecting receptacle may be used, for air and urine must traverse the same distal length of rubber tubing. If a vented receptacle is used, the set-up will not be functional because displaced air will escape through the vent in the receptacle instead of being displaced upward into the distal portion of the drainage tubing (against the downward flow of urine) and out the open arm of the glass Y tube.

Some urologists question the assumption that there is a slower rate of emptying afforded through use of the vented gravity drainage set-up. They prefer to use a low decompression drainage system, which is discussed below.

DECOMPRESSION DRAINAGE

If a patient is markedly distended or has a history of chronic urinary retention, a *decompression drainage system* may be ordered as a means of preventing total, rapid emptying of the bladder. As the name implies, the primary objective of this system is to decompress the bladder, and this is realized through an essentially *antigravity* set-up (see Fig. 7). Urine must flow against the pull of gravity, thereby prohibiting a complete emptying of the bladder during a short interval of time. When the bladder is *markedly* distended, the blood vessels as well as the musculature of the organ are stretched as a result of the increased intravesical pressure which builds up from retained urine. The rapid emptying of such a bladder— leading to a sudden withdrawal of pressure—would precipitate the rupture of some of these blood vessels and gross hematuria might well develop in such cases. Thus a gravity type of drainage system would be contraindicated. The antigravity feature of a decompression drainage system affords a gradual emptying of a distended bladder. A major advantage of this

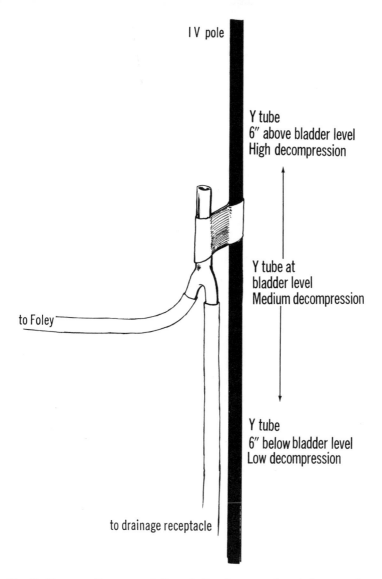

I V pole

Y tube
6″ above bladder level
High decompression

Y tube at
bladder level
Medium decompression

to Foley

Y tube
6″ below bladder level
Low decompression

to drainage receptacle

Fig. 7. Diagrammatic representation of the decompression drainage system. Note the placement of the glass Y connecting tube on the standard. The tape should not cover the bifurcation of the tube. The open arm of the Y tube allows for air to break the siphon. For high decompression, the inverted Y tube is secured to the standard at a level from 4 to 6 inches above the level of the **pubic bone.** For medium decompression, the inverted Y connecting tube is secured to the stardard **at the level of the pubic bone.** For low decompression, the inverted Y connecting tube is secured to the standard at a level which is 4 to 6 inches **below** the level of the pubic bone. Note that the pubic bone and not the bed level must be used to achieve an accurate set-up.

type of set-up is that the bladder musculature is encouraged to maintain its tone. There must be enough urine in the bladder at any given time to insure sufficient pressure to force urine upward against the pull of gravity—before it drains downward into the collecting receptacle. Through this set-up, bladder capacity is maintained. At times, the decompression drainage system is ordered for its hemostatic effect.

The antigravity feature of this system is accomplished by use of an inverted glass Y connecting tube. Latex tubing connected to the Foley catheter by a straight glass or plastic connecting tube is inserted into one of the short arms of the Y tube, and the other short arm of the Y tube is connected to a length of gravity drainage tubing which terminates in a collecting receptacle. The inverted long arm of the Y tube is left open to the air, and is secured to an IV pole or some other standard by a strip of adhesive tape (see Fig. 7). In securing the Y tube to the standard with the adhesive strip, the nurse should avoid obliterating the area of bifurcation. Observation of urinary flow up one of the short arms and down the other into the gravity drainage tubing and collecting receptacle is an essential aid in determining whether the system is functioning properly.

There are three types of decompression drainage set-ups currently used: high, medium, and low decompression drainage systems. The degree of bladder distention usually determines which type of decompression system the doctor will order and the height *above* or *below* bladder level at which the inverted Y connecting tube is taped to the standard designates the type of decompression system which will be used.

High decompression drainage may be achieved by securing the inverted Y connecting tube to the standard at a height of 4 to 6 inches above the level of the symphysis pubis (pubic bone). The height may vary from institution to institution—some doctors request the level to be as high as 8 inches above the pubic bone; however, the nurse must always remember to use the patient's *pubic bone* and not the bed level as the guide when positioning the inverted Y tube for high decompression drainage. This type of drainage system is usually ordered for the markedly distended patient whose intravesical pressure is great enough to force urine 6 inches or more upward *against* the pull of gravity before it drains downward into the collecting receptacle as the bladder is evacuated. This set-up allows for the gradual release of such pressure.

When a patient is moderately distended, *medium decompression drainage* may be ordered. For this set-up, the inverted Y connecting tube is taped to the standard at a height which is *at the level* of the pubic bone. The urine flows against the pull of gravity only the short distance up the incline of the short arm of the inverted Y tube, but this requires some degree of intravesical pressure to be sustained so that the urine may be forced upward for even this short distance.

The *low decompression drainage system* is commonly ordered for the patient presenting with a long-standing history of retention or with gross hematuria. The inverted Y tube must be secured to the standard at a level which is 4 to 6 inches *below* the level of the pubic bone to accomplish the objectives of this system. Although the downward flow of urine is interrupted by the subtle upward incline of the short arm of the inverted Y connector, even this limited antigravity flow will accomplish a more gradual emptying of the mildly distended bladder than either of the gravity drainage set-ups.

Occasionally, the doctor will write orders for the height of the inverted Y tube of a high decompression drainage system to be lowered 1 or 2 inches hourly, every 4 hours, or once per shift until the patient's bladder is completely decompressed. Then the patient is usually placed on straight gravity drainage. The nurse will know when the decompression system should be discontinued and the gravity system connected because, when the inverted Y tube connector reaches a level approximately 8 to 10 inches below the level of the symphysis, urine will flow out the open end of the inverted Y tube and spill onto the floor. This occurs because the height of the gravity portion of this system is not sufficient to sustain its function.

IRRIGATING SYSTEMS

When caring for a urologic patient with an indwelling catheter in the bladder, the nurse should remember that *routine* irrigations are not usually given. A PRN irrigation order means *only when absolutely necessary* and implies that—should the nurse note the catheter draining sluggishly—then and only then should irrigation be done. It should be remembered that the best way to keep the catheter patent and to prevent sediment from obstructing the outflow of urine is through *physiologic* irrigation, which encourages adequate fluid intake. This is one of the reasons why urologic patients are urged to force fluids to approximately 3,000 ml daily (unless contraindicated because of associated disease). However, if infection is present, the doctor may want the bladder lavaged with a medicated solution; or, if there is bleeding, the doctor may want a steady stream of solution kept running into the bladder to keep clot formation under control. Thus, for whatever reason an irrigating system is ordered, there are two such systems commonly used in the treatment of urogenital disorders: the intermittent bladder irrigation system and the constant bladder irrigation system.

In order to execute a standard bladder irrigation, the nurse must (1) disconnect the Foley catheter from the drainage system to which it is attached; (2) instill the desired irrigating solution while maintaining aseptic technique; (3) allow solution to drain from the Foley into an emesis basin; and (4) repeat the instillation and drainage procedure until the amount of solution ordered for the irrigation has been given. Should this treatment be ordered for every 2 or 3 hours during the 24-hour period, it is easy to appreciate how great the possibility of introducing infection would be—not to mention how often the patient's rest would have to be interrupted during the night. Therefore, when frequent bladder irrigations are ordered (hourly, every 2 hours, or every 3 hours), a special *closed* irrigation system may be utilized. This *intermittent bladder irrigation system* protects the patient by reducing the possibility of the introduction of infection into the bladder.

Although the three-way Foley catheter is most often used, when drainage *and* irrigation set-ups are desired, the glass Y connecting tube may again be employed to accomplish the objective of this system if a single lumen Foley is in situ. In this instance, the Y tube is positioned so that solution is allowed to flow into the bladder through one of the short arms and out of the bladder through the other (see Fig. 8). The long arm of the Y connector is attached to the Foley catheter; one of the short arms is attached—by a length of latex tubing—to the bottle containing the irrigating solution ordered, and the other short arm is attached to the desired drainage system. Two screw clamps are needed to complete the functioning of this set-up: one placed near the irrigating solution bottle on the length of latex tubing, and the other positioned close to the area of insertion of the Foley catheter on the proximal end of the length of drainage tubing. The clamp positioned near the irrigation solution bottle may remain closed to allow the bladder to be drained by the drainage system ordered. When the time comes to execute the irrigation treatment, the nurse need only tighten the clamp on the outflow (drainage) tubing and open the clamp on the inflow (irrigation) tubing. When the desired amount of solution has been allowed to flow into the bladder, the inflow clamp is tightened and the outflow clamp released. Thereafter, the bladder may be allowed to drain by the drainage system ordered until the next irrigation is due. Thus the intermittent bladder irrigation set-up serves to minimize the amount of handling of the Foley

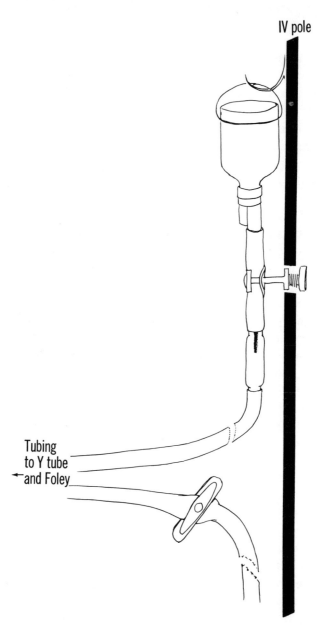

IV pole

Tubing
to Y tube
and Foley

Fig. 8. Diagrammatic representation of the intermittent bladder irrigation set-up. Note the placement of the screw clamps: one is near the irrigating solution bottle and the other is close to the area of insertion of the Foley catheter.

catheter. The nurse need only replace bottles of solution as they empty.

When frequent irrigations are ordered, this type of irrigating apparatus eliminates the need for the insertion of a three-way Foley catheter solely for the purpose of providing the patient with an irrigation system. (When a regular Foley catheter is in place, replacing it with a three-way Foley catheter would require intubation of the urethra a second time. Many urologists try to avoid this whenever possible.) However, if a three-way Foley catheter is already in place, IV tubing is usually attached to the irrigating solution bottle and then connected to the smaller irrigating arm of the catheter, while urinary drainage tubing is connected to the larger outflow (drainage) arm of the three-way Foley.

The Y tube irrigation set-up may also be utilized when a cystostomy tube is in place. It is not practical for use with nephrostomy tubes, however, because the capacity of the kidney pelvis is only 8 to 10 ml. It would be impossible to restrict inflow of the irrigating solution to such a limited amount with the apparatus described.

When carrying out the treatment, the nurse should allow no more than 120 ml of solution to enter the bladder at any given time. Since bladder capacity is approximately 500 ml, more than 60 ml may be permitted to flow into the bladder during the course of an irrigation. However, it should be noted that the irrigating solution is flowing downward from a bottle suspended approximately 3 feet above the bladder. Most patients will experience mild discomfort when amounts greater than 120 ml are allowed to flow in. Increased irritability of the bladder musculature subsequent to bacterial invasion or pathologic changes accounts for much of this discomfort.

The set-up for the *constant bladder irrigation* (sometimes referred to as a "through and through" set-up) is essentially the same as for the intermittent bladder irrigation except that, since solution will be flowing into the bladder constantly, there is a drip regulator positioned immediately below the clamp adjacent to the solution bottle. The doctor will order the desired irrigating solution, but frequently will not specify the rate of flow at which it should enter the bladder. The usual rate is between 45 and 60 drops per minute, and this flow rate can be regulated with the clamp. If the apparatus described previously is used, then the outflow or drainage system should be *medium decompression drainage;* if a straight gravity drainage system is used, the constant flow from the irrigating solution will run down into the collecting receptacle of the drainage system and *not* into the bladder, thus making the system nonfunctional. With the outflow to medium decompression, however, the bladder will have to retain solution until there is enough intravesical pressure to force the fluid against gravity up the short arm of the Y tube of this setup before flowing down into the drainage collecting receptacle. If a three-way Foley catheter is in place, the outflow may be to either of the aforementioned gravity systems of drainage, as the unique inflow channel of this catheter insures entrance of the irrigating solution into the bladder.

The constant bladder irrigation system is most often used after transurethral prostatectomy as a means of combating the oozing (and resultant clot formation) from the venous sinus of the prostatic bed. It is also utilized when topical administration of medication is ordered to treat an acute inflammatory process of the bladder.

NURSING RESPONSIBILITIES

The nursing student has specific responsibilities for the implementation and maintenance of urinary tract drainage and irrigating apparatus. The drainage or irrigating system that the doctor orders must be set up properly, and this entails understanding of the underlying functional principles inherent in the system as well as knowledge of the dynamics of the system itself. Once the system is operational, proper maintenance is most important. Observation may be done systematically if the student will begin by checking the area closest to the patient and then work downward or upward as circumstances warrant.

When securing tubing to the bed, the student should take care not to obstruct the lumen of the drainage tubing. A "spring clip" or pin attached to a tape-tab or a looped rubber band is more desirable than placement of a pin directly around the tubing itself. A pin placed around the tubing itself depresses the lumen and often forces the tubing to bend on itself, thereby blocking the free outward flow of the urinary drainage. The tape or rubber band tab helps to prevent the tubing from twisting or kinking. The student should also observe the drainage tubing to make sure that it is always positioned *over* the thigh. This precaution prevents the clamping off of the tube by the weight of the body pressing on it and lessens the danger of pressure sores for the patient who is on bedrest. It must be remembered that the skin of patients in the older age group is predisposed to the formation of pressure areas.

To insure that the tubing is patent, the student should observe the amount of drainage present in the collecting receptacle. If the level of drainage in the collection receptacle has not changed over a period of hours, the patient should be encouraged to force fluids within a concentrated period of time. In an hours time thereafter, if the flow still seems sluggish, the catheter should be irrigated. If there is no order for a PRN irrigation, the doctor should be notified and an order obtained.

The changing (if plastic is used) or cleansing (if glass is used) of the drainage receptacle at least once each day completes the maintenance of the system, and will help to keep odor to a minimum.

In conclusion, the student should remember the importance of the accurate recording of intake and output for the urologic patient. This balance is of specific importance to the doctor when further treatment is being planned and when the patient's physical status is being evaluated. When an irrigating system is employed, the nurse must carefully record the amount of solution which has been allowed to flow into the bladder during the course of the treatments that are given on each shift. When the 8-hour totals are recorded, these amounts must be subtracted from the total urinary drainage in the collecting receptacle to give the correct picture of the patient's urinary output.

REFERENCES

1. Creevy, C. D. Outline of Urology, New York, Blakiston Division, McGraw-Hill Book Company, 1964.
2. Hamm, F. C., and Weinberg, S. R. Urology in Medical Practice, 2nd ed. Philadelphia, J. B. Lippincott Co., 1962.
3. Marshall, V. F. Textbook of Urology, 2nd ed. New York, Hoeber Medical Division, Harper & Row, Publishers, 1964.

4

Infectious Conditions of the Urogenital Tract

For the purposes of this text, the care of urologic patients presenting with those categories of conditions most frequently encountered by the nurse will be discussed. Anomalies and other conditions less frequently encountered are interesting physiologic phenomena, but they may be researched as they present themselves: the data being added to that base of fundamental knowledge necessary for sound nursing practice. Since the inflammatory processes seen in the urogenital tract are most frequently secondary to the entrance of pathogenic organisms, nursing care of the patient with an infection of the urogenital tract will be elaborated.

The student should be cautioned to avoid a reporting and recording error which commonly occurs. Clarification of terminology is always indicated so that students are encouraged to use correct terms when describing diseases of their patients. Although the terms *inflammation* and *infection* are often used interchangeably when disease processes are being described, an *inflammatory process* is one that may evolve as the result of tissue reaction to chemical, bacterial, manipulative, or toxic irritation while pathogenic microorganisms are the sole initiators of an *infectious process*. Thus inflammatory conditions of the urogenital tract may occur *without* infection, and it should be evident that the interchangeable use of the terms *inflammatory* and *infectious* is erroneous unless there are laboratory data to substantiate the assumption (inherent in the terms' interchangeable use) that an inflammatory process is indeed associated with an infection.

It should also be mentioned that varied pathogenesis, symptomatology, and prognosis render infectious disease processes of the urogenital tract difficult to elaborate. Therefore, for the sake of clarity, this chapter will be divided into two sections: Care of the Patient with Urinary-Tract Infection, and Care of the Male Patient with Genital-Tract Infection. As mentioned in the preface, inflammatory and infectious conditions of the female genital system will not be discussed in this text because this topic is covered in gynecology books and is most often discussed at length during the student's course in obstetrics. However, since the urinary system of the male is essentially the same as that of the female, the discussion of infection of that tract will be generally applicable to both male and female patients.

CARE OF THE PATIENT WITH URINARY-TRACT INFECTION

It is generally agreed that only respiratory infections occur more frequently than infections of the urinary tract. Such infections occur most frequently in children of both sexes, in women who are of child-bearing age, and in the elderly of both sexes. Urinary-tract infections are seldom seen in younger adult males—the majority of episodes of infection in men occur after the age of 40—while these infections are about three times more common in women. Within the adult female population, urinary-tract infections occur more frequently in pregnant than in nonpregnant women; and, except for excessive weight gain, pyelonephritis is probably the most common complication of pregnancy. Infection of the urinary tract may also follow a single catheterization of a patient, and almost all patients who have catheters indwelling for a period exceeding three days (regardless of whether antibacterial prophylaxis is implemented) develop such infection.

At this juncture, the reader should be urged to remember that—*regardless of the specific disease entity*—the generative focus of this chapter is the infectious process; and one of the most important principles underlying any disease of this process is that the various infectious diseases of the urinary tract are caused by the *same strains* of infecting organisms. Increasingly, it is being established that most of the causative bacteria of urinary-tract infections originate in the intestinal tract of the host—some strains of *Pseudomonas* and *Staphylococcus* being the only exceptions; *Escherichia coli* has been found to be the most common pathogen (Seneca et al., 1964). The five most frequent causative organisms of urinary-tract infection are *E. coli*, *Proteus*, *Pseudomonas*, *Streptococci*, and *Staphylococci* (Martin and Wagoner, 1965a).

Another important fact to be remembered is that the main objectives of nursing care for the patient with an infection of the urinary tract are prevention of superimposed infection, implementation of the medical plan for the eradication of the existing infection, and relief of the patient's discomfort. Infection in the urinary tract is particularly undesirable because damage to renal tissue may result; thus the nurse should be acutely aware of the importance of early detection as an invaluable aid in the prevention of significant renal impairment. Although the ability to recognize signs and symptoms of such infection expedite early detection, the primary concerns of the student are problem-solving in nursing intervention to encourage the distressed individual to seek medical assist-

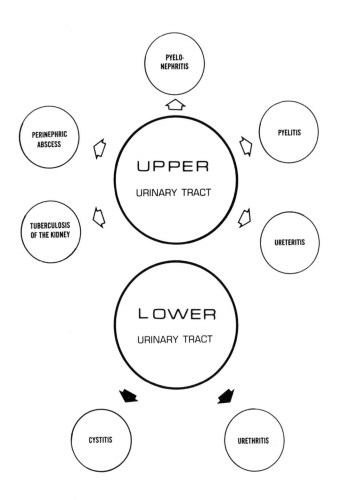

Fig. 1. Infections of the upper and lower urinary tract. The infections have been grouped in this manner so that an association may be made between specific disease entities and area of occurrence. The most common manifestations of infections of the upper urinary tract are complaints of chills, fever, pain, and/or tenderness in the flank and generalized malaise. **Hematuria is not characteristic of infections in this area.** The most common manifestations of infections of the lower urinary tract are complaints of frequency, urgency, dysuria, and/or burning on urination. **Burning on urination does not always indicate infection;** other disease processes may cause this symptom.

ance, and—after the individual has been seen by the doctor and a plan for medical diagnosis and treatment has been formulated—the development and implementation of a nursing-care plan. Lengthy discussion of specific disease entities (as outlined in Fig. 1) will, therefore, be omitted. Interested students may review the references listed at the end of the chapter. The ensuing discussion will be focused on clinical manifestations of infections of the urinary tract and on indications for nursing care in managing these disorders.

When thinking of the etiology of urinary-tract infections, the student should be aware of the roles played by anatomic and bacteriologic factors. Anatomic considerations should include thoughts about *where* the infection is (upper or lower tract) and *what* route of entry the infecting organism might have taken. Bacteriologic considerations should include consideration of the causative organism or organisms. These are the intellectual-processes crucial to the development of appropriate nursing behavior; they facilitate the problem-solving approaches that will lead to meaningful nursing care for the patient with a urinary-tract infection.

It is generally agreed that the most common predisposing factor of urinary-tract infection is obstruction to the free flow of urine anywhere between the substance of the kidneys (kidney parenchyma) and the urethral outlet. Such obstruction results in poor drainage of urine and may cause varying degrees of dilatation of the bladder, leading to trabeculation (sagging of atonic mucous membrane between overworked hypertrophied muscle bands of the bladder) and hypertrophy (see Fig. 2). Obstructive lesions may be structural or functional, acquired or congenital. Stasis of urine secondary to such obstruction and/or reflux of urine from the bladder into the ureters encourages the growth and transfer of pathogenic organisms. Other predisposing factors include anatomc lesions within the tract, and the presence of a foreign body in the renal pelvis or bladder—most commonly a calculus. Since the

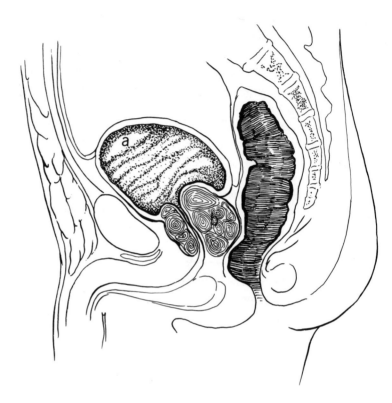

Fig. 2. Obstruction at the bladder neck as caused by prostatic hypertrophy (b). The wrinkles within the bladder wall are called **trabeculations** (a).

aforementioned conditions often tend to perpetuate chronic infections, the patient may require surgical intervention to eradicate such secondary infectious processes.

Acute infections of the tract are usually manifested by fever accompanying the local symptoms of pain and/or discomfort. Such infections—commonly seen in young or middle-aged women—are not usually associated with detectable predisposing disease; they tend to be self-limiting, and usually respond to minimal medical treatment. If there is pain or tenderness in the flank the infection usually involves the upper tract (see Fig. 1). This can be easily understood when the student recalls that the kidneys and upper two-thirds of the ureters are located within the costovertebral angle (CVA). When speaking of the *flank*, the nurse is referring to the area of the body known as the patient's side—between the ribs and the hips. In most of these acute infections it may be noted that local and constitutional symptoms are in direct relation to the severity of the urinary infection (Martin and Wagoner, 1965a). Pain or tenderness localized in the suprapubic and perineal regions suggest involvement of the lower urinary tract; and, again, there is a direct relationship between the site of the pain and the anatomic location of the lower third of the ureters, the bladder, and the urethra. In contrast to simple states of acute infection which tend to be self-limiting, there are more serious states such as renal abscess that may be associated with bacteremia or endocarditis.

Recurrent infection of the urinary tract is often difficult to distinguish from chronic states of infection. However, unlike acute or recurrent infections, predisposing disease is often present in the chronic infectious states. Chronic infections of the urinary tract are often asymptomatic. When a patient manifests none of the symptoms of urinary-tract infection, but demonstrates a significant urinary bacterial count, he is said to have *asymptomatic bacteriuria*. At times, however, chronic infectious processes produce recurrent or continuous symptoms. These symptoms may vary from ones that are annoying and mildly distressing (e.g., polyuria or nocturia) to complaints of flank pain, fever, chills, and/or dysuria. Sometimes, manifestations are more nonspecific, and the patient may only complain of fatigue or intermittent low backache. Investigation of the urinary tract is usually considered when no other explanation for loss of weight, anemia, persistent nausea and vomiting, hypertension, and fever can be determined.

The laboratory findings in chronic disease include proteinuria, abnormal urinary sediment, and azotemia. These findings reflect the renal damage present and the resultant impaired function. Further, chronic infection is characterized by an insidious onset; there may be no previous history of urinary infection. Thus chronic states do *not* necessarily result from preceding acute infections. Laboratory findings of bacteriuria (and almost always pyuria) are still the most conclusive evidence in the diagnosis of urinary-tract infection. A bacterial count of 100,000 or more organisms per milliliter of urine is considered true bacteriuria. As previously mentioned, the most common organism isolated from patients with significant bacteriuria is *Escherichia coli* (Patton and Ross, 1967), which causes 42 percent of the lower tract infections and 51 percent of the cases of chronic pyelonephritis (Seneca et al., 1964; Smith and Martin, 1966). However, other pathogens are also believed to have an influence on the infectious process. These include viruses and/or immunologic reaction to specific baterial antigens (or to an antigen of renal origin released or altered by infection) which could produce the clinical manifestations of chronic pyelonephritis (Stamey et al., 1965).

Albuminuria is a common finding in patients with chronic urinary-tract infection, and may amount to as much as 2 g per 24 hours in some cases. If additional renal disease is present, microscopic examination may reveal even higher values. *Pyuria*, rarely absent in *acute* urinary-tract infections, appears less frequently in cases of asymptomatic bacteriuria and the various kinds of *chronic* urinary-tract infection. However, as it is commonly found in other forms of genitourinary-tract disorders, pyuria alone is not a definite index of urinary-tract infection. In other diseases of the kidney, *casts of leukocytes* may also be observed, but these structures are *not* characteristic of infectious processes in the upper urinary tract. Renal biopsy has been employed to corroborate a tentative diagnosis of upper urinary-tract infection. This technique has met with varying success (Brumfitt and Percival, 1962; Gonder, 1965; Jackson et al., 1957; and Seneca and Peer, 1965) and, currently, changes in renal tissue are ascribed to an infectious process *only* if the biopsy material revealing an interstitial inflammatory process also yields a positive bacterial culture. Thus it may be said that bacteriologic findings are the basis for a diagnosis of urinary-tract infection.

The route taken by organisms which tend to infect the urinary tract is still being debated by urologists, and remains essentially unknown. However, most clinical evidence points to two routes of entry: (1) the hematologic or descending route—the blood stream being the mode of transportation for the infecting organisms, and (2) the ascending route—the urethra being the portal of entry with organisms traveling upward in the tract. The hematologic route is usually secondary to infection elsewhere in the body, and the nurse can only hope to implement the care plan efficiently so that further deterioration of renal function may be prevented and the symptoms alleviated. To prevent primary infection of the urinary tract, however, teaching the patient is again the best precautionary measure. Since it is known that organisms of the intestinal tract are the chief culprits of urinary-tract infection, the importance after defecation of directing tissue paper *from* the area of the labia downward and backward rather than from the perianal area upward should be impressed upon patients. Cleansing from the perianal area upward toward the area of the urinary meatus increases the possibility of contamination of that orifice with the principle infecting organism from the intestinal tract (*E. coli*).

To minimize the incidence of infection secondary to intubation of the urinary tract, proper preparation of the patient prior to catheterization is essential; contamination may occur when the catheter is passed through the urethra if the surrounding area has not been properly cleansed. It should be remembered, however, that normally the urinary tract has considerable resistance to infection and instrumentation may be done without causing infection. But the urologic patient is more likely *not* to have a normal urinary tract, so this patient tends to be predisposed to infection. Regardless of the infectious potential of instruments or catheters, the benefit of their use in the urologic patient is indisputable. Nursing responsibility after catheterization (or instrumentation) involves observation of the vital signs—*temperature* being of most importance—and the forcing of fluids (within the limits of the patient's renal function) to insure *internal* or *physiologic irrigation* of the urinary tract.

There are a group of signs and symptoms which are characteristic of urinary-tract infection and which serve to alert the medical and nursing staff of the possibility of such an infectious process. The most common clinical manifestations of an infection of the *upper urinary tract* are complaints of chills, fever, pain, and/or tenderness in the flank, and generalized malaise. Hematuria is *not* characteristic of pyelonephritis; tumors or other lesions are usually responsible for this occurrence. When there is infection in the *lower urinary tract*, the patient will usually complain of frequency and/or urgency of urination, dysuria, and burning on urination. Burning on urination does not always indicate infection, however; other noninfectious processes may produce this sensation.

Since findings of bacteriuria give conclusive proof of urinary-tract infection, it may be clearly understood why the proper techniques for collection of the urine specimen for bacteriologic culture are such important responsibilities of the nurse. Collection of a midstream-voided specimen after the glans has been cleansed is usually adequate for male patients. In the female patient, however, a catheterized specimen is usually preferable. Midstream specimens from female patients are often not free of contaminants because of excessive vaginal secretions or urine passing over the labia unavoidably. Also, female patients often complain of being unable to void when the labia are held apart to effect separation for the mid-stream specimen. Thus the catheterized specimen will minimize the chances of contamination, and the nurse must adhere to the principles of asepsis during catheterization to minimize the chances of superimposed infection.

Transportation of the urine specimen is also an important responsibility of the nurse. The reader may question the inclusion of this function as a nursing responsibility, but attention to details like these facilitates the diagnosis and treatment of the patient. When a urine specimen for culture is allowed to remain at room temperature for more than 1 hour, or in a refrigerator for longer than 24 hours, it is not suitable for quantitative culture analysis. Studies carried out on such a specimen often yield inaccurate results, thereby necessitating collection of other specimens. When this occurs, time is wasted and unnecessary expense is incurred by the patient. Therefore, the nurse should make arrangements for or supervise the immediate refrigeration (or rapid transportation) of the specimen to the laboratory for microbiologic study. It is also advisable for ancillary personnel to be made aware of the importance of such specimens reaching the laboratory as soon as possible after their collection.

Once a diagnosis of urinary-tract infection has been made, the nursing-care triad for patients with such a diagnosis should be implemented. The patient should be made to *force fluids* (within the limits of renal function) and *limit activity* (often being allowed out of bed, but with restrictions), while the nurse carefully *observes the urine* (see Fig. 3).

The appearance of the urine should be observed *and* recorded before the student considers an assignment completed. This should be done *in addition to* the recording of the output, because the description of visible changes in the color, amount, and quality of the urinary sedimentation are important indices of the patient's progress. When this is recorded in the nurses' notes *and* verbally communicated during the nursing report, a more complete picture of the patient's condition is obtained.

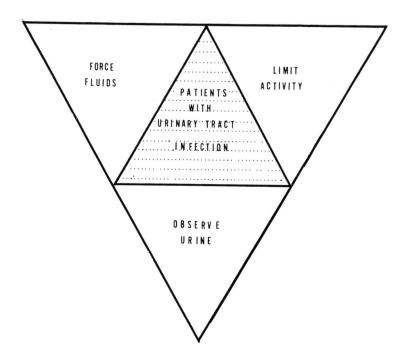

Fig. 3. The nursing care triad for patients with urinary-tract infection.

Avoidance of unnecessary urinary-tract instrumentation is also an important factor in the management of patients with urinary-tract infection, but when instrumentation is indicated, the nurse should observe for fever subsequent to that treatment and should anticipate that *both* the urine and the blood will be cultured shortly thereafter. Treatment also usually includes the prescribing of one or more antibacterial drugs given in dosages sufficient to achieve bacteriocidal or bacteriostatic levels. Use of specific therapeutic agents varies from doctor to doctor and from institution to institution; but, whatever drug is ordered for the patient, it is the responsibility of the nurse to know the *untoward effects* of that drug as well as the dosage to be given. It is with this total comprehension that meaningful nursing care may be given—and *observation* is a primary nursing activity.

CARE OF THE MALE PATIENT WITH GENITAL-TRACT INFECTION

Anatomy of the Male Genital Tract

A brief review of the anatomy and physiology of the male genital tract and its proximity to the urinary tract is in order before a discussion of infections is initiated. The male reproductive system is comprised of organs, tubular structures, glands, and supportive structures much the same as the female reproductive system. However, in addition to the functional differences, a unique characteristic of the male reproductive system is its intimate relationship to the urinary system (see Fig. 4).

The scrotum is a pendulous sac situated posterior to the penis and anterior to the anus; its tissues are continuous with those of the groin and perineum. It contains and supports the testes—paired, oval shaped, glandular organs. It also contains the epididymides and the proximal portions of the spermatic cords—the vas deferens and the testicular vessels. The scrotum is divided into right and left compartments by a septum, and each compartment contains a testis; the left compartment hangs lower than the right because of the longer spermatic cord of the left testicle. The wall of the scrotum is comprised of skin and a fascial layer of connective tissue that contains smooth muscle fibers; lining the inner surface of this layer is the parietal layer of the tunica vaginalis.

The testes produce the male germ cell and the male hormones. Each is surrounded by a capsule of fibrous tissue, the tunica albuginea; from the inner surface of this capsule, con-

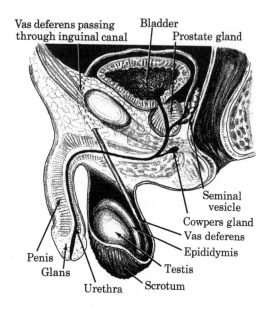

Fig. 4. The male urinary and reproductive systems. (From Dawson. Basic Human Anatomy. 1966. Courtesy of Appleton-Century-Crofts.)

nective tissue septa extend into the body of the testis dividing it into lobules. The seminiferous tubules are located within the lobules of the testes, and the cells within these tubules produce the male germ cells. The seminiferous tubules are supported and surrounded by loose connective tissue, and this connective tissue contains interstitial cells which produce the male hormone.

The epididymis is an elongated excretory duct which is located on the posterolateral surface of each testis. Its proximal portion firmly articulates with the testis and precedes the tortuously coiled, tubular portion—approximately 4 cm in length —which comprises the body of the structure. The distal portion of the epididymis is less convoluted and tapers to become the vas (ductus) deferens; thus, the epididymis may be thought of as being the convoluted beginning of the vas deferens.

The vas deferens is a long tubular structure which extends from the epididymis to the ejaculatory duct. It is a component of the spermatic cord and is held in proximity to the veins, arteries, lymphatic vessels, and nerves of that cord by connective tissue. The vas deferens rises out of the scrotum and then traverses the inguinal canal as part of the spermatic cord. After it enters the abdominal cavity, it leaves the other cord structures and terminates near the base of the prostate gland as the ejaculatory duct (having joined the duct of the seminal vesicle immediately prior to termination). The vas deferens expedites the passage of sperm.

The paired seminal vesicles, like the prostate gland and bulbourethral (Cowper's) glands, are accessory glands of the male reproductive system. They are pyramidal shaped and are located above the prostate gland in an area between the bladder and the rectum. They secrete a sticky, yellowish, alkaline fluid which provides nutrient substance for the sperm and produces most of the secretion for the semen. The seminal ducts join with the vas deferens and form the ejaculatory ducts; the ejaculatory ducts then traverse the prostate gland to unite with the prostatic part of the urethra. They convey the semen to the urethra.

The bulbourethral (Cowper's) glands—located on either side of the membranous urethra—secrete a thick, sticky, alkaline fluid which adds to the semen and is believed to assist in neutralizing the acid environment of the vagina. The prostate gland lies anterior to the rectum and just below the neck of the bladder surrounding the proximal portion of the urethra. It secretes a thin, alkaline fluid which is also added to the semen; however, in addition, prostatic fluid in small amounts continually empties through ducts into the posterior urethra (from 0.5 to 2 ml per hour), and in much larger amounts during coitus. Secretions from both of these glands are believed to enhance the vitality of the sperm.

The penis is traversed through its length by the urethra,

which is composed of three segments: the prostatic urethra, the membranous urethra, and the cavernous (penile) urethra. In the male, the urethra serves as a passageway for the reproductive *and* the urinary system.

Nursing Considerations

Inflammation of the urethra (urethritis) may occur secondary to nonspecific gonorrheal or tuberculous bacterial invasion. The patient is usually in acute distress as he may experience burning on urination, frequency, urgency, and/or dysuria. Broad-spectrum antibiotics are usually ordered, and the student should encourage the patient to rest and to force fluids. If there is a discharge from the urethra, meticulous handwashing after contact with the genitals should be encouraged in the patient. On some units the linens and towels are treated like contaminated bedclothes and as such are placed in a special laundry bag. If the patient is at home, he should be encouraged to keep his linens, clothing, washcloths, and towels separated from those of the rest of the family until the infectious process has been successfully treated. He should also be advised against having intercourse as this would lead to transmission of the infection. Sitz or tub baths tend to be soothing for the patient. The surrounding area should be cleansed periodically during the day.

Prostatitis (an inflammation of the prostate gland) may be a direct extension of infections of the bladder or urethra, or caused by blood- or lymph-borne organisms from infections elsewhere in the body. Young adult males and older men are commonly seen to present with this condition. Although the condition is often asymptomatic, patients may complain of frequent, painful, or difficult voiding, and perineal tenderness and pain, fever, and/or malaise. The medical management is usually conservative: gentle prostatic massage (accomplished by the introduction of a gloved finger into the rectum) will tend to empty the prostate and vesicles, resulting in relief for the patient. Usually the patient is to be encouraged to force fluids and to rest. When local application of heat is desired, warm sitz baths are usually ordered. Antibiotics and other chemotherapeutic agents may also be ordered. The student's primary responsibility, however, will be to insure that the patient's activity is limited and that he forces fluids.

When an infection passes up through the urethra and ejaculatory duct and along the vas deferens, epididymitis usually results (see Fig. 5). It often occurs secondary to prostatitis or infection of the seminal vesicles, and is probably the most common of all scrotal lesions. The testis of the affected side is rarely involved initially. The patient usually complains of a pain and/or soreness in the groin. Pain and swelling in the scrotum may develop thereafter, and the patient may become febrile. Again, the forcing of fluids (at least 3,000 ml daily) to keep the body adequately hydrated is of utmost importance, and the scrotum is usually elevated to prevent tension on the spermatic cord. Such elevation may be accomplished with a modified version of the Bellevue bridge (see Fig. 6). A long (27 inches or more if necessary) strip of 3-inch adhesive tape with a 6- to 8-inch strip superimposed at its center may be positioned on the patient after tincture of benzoin has been applied to his skin in the area of the two hip bones, in front and laterally. Tincture of benzoin should be applied only in amounts sufficient to accommodate the 3-inch width of the tape; it is not necessary to paint the entire abdominal, pelvic, and lower-back region because in this instance the sole function of the solution is to protect the skin and to enhance the sticking potential of the adhesive. The patient may be instructed to place an abdominal pad (combine) between the central portion of the bridge and the scrotum, thereby providing a cushioned surface for his added comfort. With this modified Bellevue bridge in place, the patient is afforded mobility and sup-

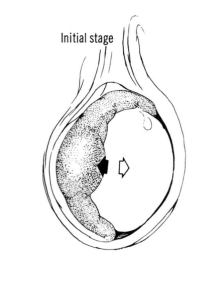

Initial stage

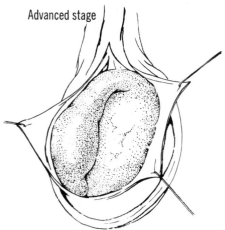

Advanced stage

Fig. 5. Acute epididymitis. Note the swelling of the epididymis. In the initial stages of the disease, congestion of the testicle may be noted; but the testicle will not be swollen or tender. (The dark arrow is pointing to the swollen epididymis. The white arrow is pointing to the congested testicle.) In the advanced stage, there is swelling and tenderness of **both** epididymis and testicle.

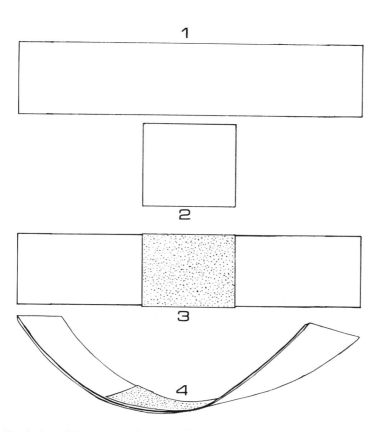

Fig. 6. A modified version of the Bellevue Bridge. 1. A strip of adhesive tape 3 inches in width and 27 inches or more in length. 2. A strip of adhesive tape 3 inches in width and 6–8 inches in length. 3. The smaller length of tape is superimposed on the center of the longer length. 4. The bridge or sling is ready to be placed under the scrotum and positioned on the skin area above the two hip bones in front and laterally.

port whether he is in the supine or upright position. Local application of ice may also be ordered to reduce the swelling and to relieve the pain. A rubber glove filled with ice is particularly suitable for such an application because the palm area may be placed under the scrotum while the finger areas are placed on either side of the scrotum. If an ice cap is used, it should be placed *under* the scrotum. It is flexible and not bulky, but should be removed periodically to prevent damage to the skin of the scrotum. Local application of heat is usually contraindicated because of the proximity of the testes, which require an environment cooler than body temperature for the survival of the germinal cells they contain.

Orchitis (inflammation of the testes) may result from systemic infection, but the mumps virus is probably the most common cause of acute orchitis (see Fig. 7). If parotitis (inflammation of the parotid gland) precedes the testicular swelling, orchitis is suspected. The testicle usually becomes swollen, tense, and painful, and the scrotum is reddened and edematous. The patient also has an elevated temperature. The patient may appear acutely ill and complain of nausea and vomiting or of other systemic symptoms such as chills. The sudden cessation of pain is a danger signal that the marked swelling of the testicle may have shut off the blood supply to that organ. Treatment is usually conservative, with the patient on bedrest. The scrotum should be elevated, and local application of ice may be instituted. The patient's fluid intake is usually increased to 3,000 ml or more per day. If pus formation (suppuration) occurs, incision and drainage may be necessary; or surgical opening of the tunica albuginea may be indicated if circulation is impaired.

Although the etiology of chronic hydrocele is unknown, the general category *hydrocele* will be included at this juncture because acute cases may occur secondary to acute epididymitis or orchitis, and swelling of the scrotum is manifested. Unlike inflammatory processes in general, *no pain* is associated with hydrocele. However, on occasion it becomes so large that the patient experiences a dragging or dull aching sensation in the scrotum or groin. Hydrocele is defined as a collection of fluid within the tunica vaginalis that surrounds the testicle. The fluid is usually clear, amber, or yellow, and it collects about the testicle. The mass grows gradually; it may be a soft,

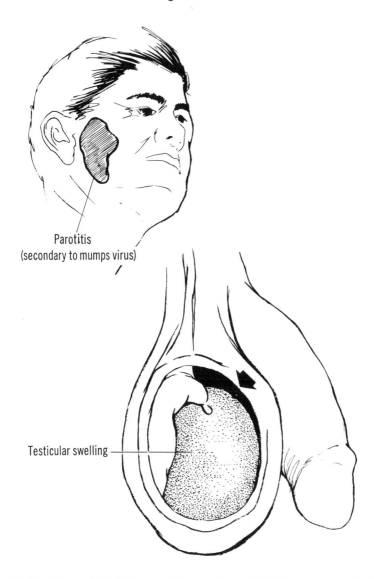

Fig. 7. Acute orchitis. When parotitis precedes a testicular swelling, orchitis secondary to the mumps virus is suspected. The testicle is usually enlarged and tender and tense to the touch. The scrotum appears reddened and edematous. A secondary hydrocele may develop (note arrow).

cystic mass, or it may become so tense that it simulates a solid tumor. When a differential diagnosis is to be made, the transillumination procedure (see Fig. 8) is often indicated. In a completely darkened room, a flashlight with a bright beam is positioned firmly against the wall of the scrotum. If the light shows through the scrotum, a hydrocele is present. It should be noted, however, that a hydrocele may be present with a tumor mass. The tumor will *not* transilluminate.

Although hydrocelectomy is usually defined as the excision of the tunica vaginalis, there are methods of hydroce-

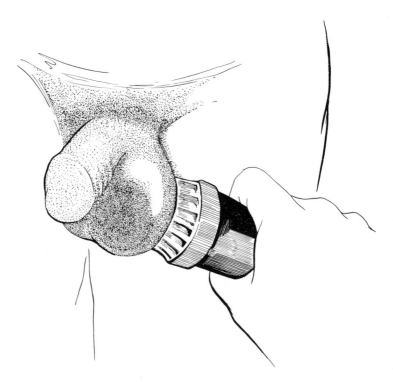

Fig. 8. Transillumination of the scrotum. This is accomplished when a flashlight with a bright beam is positioned firmly against the wall of the scrotum. Note that the light shows through the scrotum. This indicates the presence of fluid and not a tumor mass.

lectomy which do not require excision of the tunica vaginalis. Hydrocelectomy is the preferred treatment when a very tense hydrocele impairs circulation to the testes or when a bulky mass proves uncomfortable to the patient. The postoperative course is usually uneventful, and the student must remember to change dressings once such change is permitted by the doctor. The embarrassment of the patient is usually the central problem to be solved. When proper draping procedure is followed and the patient's privacy is secured, this reaction may be greatly minimized. Some urologists aspirate the fluid from the scrotum, and occasionally a drain may be left in place. Seepage requires frequent dressing changes, and—if the patient is provided with combines (abdominal pads) and instructed as to how the dressing is to be done—*he* will be able to do it.

In such cases, the nurse should observe the affected area at least once per shift to insure its cleanliness and to be able to report its condition. The color, amount, and consistency of the exudate should also be noted, recorded, and reported. Even when a patient changes his own dressings, the responsibility for the manner in which that treatment is done and the recording of the condition of the patient and his progress remains with the nurse.

REFERENCES

1. Best, C. H., and Taylor, N. B. The Physiological Basis of Medical Practice, 8th ed. Baltimore, The Williams & Wilkins Co., 1966, pp. 1649–1658.
2. Brumfitt, W., and Percival, A. Adjustment of urine pH in the chemotherapy of urinary tract infections. Lancet, 1:186–190, 1962.
3. Brun, C., et al. Simultaneous bacteriologic studies of renal biopsies and urine. *In* Kass, L. H., ed. Progress in Pyelonephritis. Philadelphia, F. A. Davis, Co., 1965.

4. Cook, E. N. Infections of the urinary tract: Fundamental concepts of diagnosis and treatment. J.A.M.A., 195:193–194, 1966.
5. Council on Drugs: A New Antibacterial Agent for Infections of the Genitourinary Tract: Neg Gram. J.A.M.A., 192:628–629, 1965.
6. Culp, D. A. Diagnostic procedures in uropediatric problems. Postgrad. Med., 33:386–394, 1963.
7. Finland, M. The present status of the chemotherapy of pyelonephritis. *In* Quinn, E. L., and Kass, E. H., eds. Biology of Pyelonephritis. Boston, Little, Brown and Company, 1960.
8. Gonder, M. J. Prostatitis. Surg. Clin. N. Amer., 45: 1449–1454, 1965.
9. Jackson, G. G., et al. Concepts of pyelonephritis: Experience with renal biopsies and long-term clinical observations. Ann. Intern. Med., 47:1165–1183, 1957.
10. Jacobson, M. H., and Newman, W. Study of pyelonephritis using renal biopsy material. Arch. Intern. Med. (Chicago), 110:211–217, 1962.
11. Kleeman, C. R., et al. Pyelonephritis. Medicine, 39:3–116, 1960.
12. Martin, W. J., and Wagoner, R. D. Infections of the urinary tract. I. Some nosologic and etiologic considerations. Minn. Med., 48:95–99, 1965a.
13. ———— and Wagoner, R. D. Infections of the urinary tract. III. Symptomatology. Minn. Med., 48:379–382, 1965b.
14. ———— and Wagoner, R. D. Infections of the urinary tract. IV. Antibacterial regimens. Minn. Med., 48:503–507, 1965c.
15. McCabe, W. R., and Jackson, G. G. Treatment of pyelonephritis: Bacterial, drug, and host factors in success or failure among 252 patients. New Eng. J. Med., 272:1037–1044, 1965.
16. McDonald, D. F., and Murphy, G. P. Bacteriostatic and acidifying effects of methionine, hydrolyzed casein, and ascorbic acid on the urine. New Eng. J. Med., 261:803–805, 1959.
17. McGeachie, J. Quantitative bacteriology of urinary infection. Brit. J. Urol., 38:294–301, 1966.
18. Patton, J. F., and Ross, G. The painful testicle. Hosp. Med., 3:24–40, (June) 1967.
19. Pawlowski, J. M., et al. Chronic pyelonephritis: A morphologic and bacteriologic study. New Eng. J. Med., 268:965–969, 1963.
20. Seneca, H., and Peer, P. Clinical laboratory diagnosis of urinary tract infections. J. Urol., 94:78–81, 1965.

21. ———— et al. The relationship among normal intestinal flora, kidney infections, and kidney stones. J. Urol., 92:603–613, 1964.
22. Smith, L. H., and Martin, W. J. Infections of the urinary tract. Med. Clin. N. Amer., 50:1127–1135, 1966.
23. Stamey, T. A., et al. The localization and treatment of urinary tract infections: The role of bactericidal urine levels as opposed to serum levels. Medicine, 44:1–36, 1965.
24. Turck, M., et al. Failure of prolonged treatment of chronic urinary-tract infections with antibiotics. New Eng. J. Med., 267:999–1005, 1962.

5

Calculi and Calculous Disease

The formation of calculi (lithiasis or the condition of having "stones") is one of the most common disease conditions of the urinary tract. It is seen more frequently in men than in women, and is a rare occurrence in children. Calculi are not likely to cause injury or symptoms if they do not obstruct urinary passages such as the UP or UV junctions. However, if they are obstructive, severe symptoms and/or renal damage may result. Another characteristic of stones is that they tend to recur. Therefore, an attempt is usually made to discover the etiology of the initial episode as a means of preventing subsequent stone formation. Calculi most commonly originate in the calyces of the kidney, but they may also be found in the bladder and occasionally within the prostate gland. When formed in the bladder, they usually are a secondary complication of some other urologic disease—the result of an obstructive lesion such as benign prostatic hypertrophy, bladder tumor, bladder neck contracture, urethral stricture; or of a bladder divericulum; or as the result of an infection. Foreign bodies in the bladder, such as catheters or other drains, may also lead to calculus formation.

The most common cause of *bladder calculus formation* is infection of residual urine with urea-splitting organisms. These organisms cause the urine to develop a strongly alkaline pH; and since calcium phosphate salts will not dissolve in alkaline urine, they are often found to be the elements of which urinary calculi of the bladder are composed. Stones found in the prostate gland are usually discovered when benign hyperthrophy of that gland is under investigation. They are rare and of little importance clinically because they cause no symptoms and no damage to surrounding tissue. Stones found in the ureter rarely originate there unless they are secondary to congenital abnormalities or acquired strictures of that structure. Ureteral stones have usually traveled downward from the kidney pelvis.

Urinary calculi fall into three categories: silent or fixed stones, free stones, and staghorn stones. Each type characteristically initiates a particular set of symptoms. The *fixed* or *silent* stone is usually found *within* or *adhering to* the kidney parenchyma. The patient is usually asymptomatic unless the growth of the stone blocks urinary flow from one of the calyces at the lower pole of the kidney. When this does occur, however, the patient usually experiences flank pain or symptoms of upper urinary-tract infection (see Chapter 4). The *free stone* is *unattached* to tissue *surfaces* and therefore is free to travel downward within the urinary tract. The patient experiences severe pain—the explanation for which varies. Some authorities believe that ureteral spasm occurs because of trauma or irritation to the walls of the ureter as the free stone is pushed downward by the peristaltic waves of that ureter. Others believe that the pain is the result of obstruction of urinary passages as the stone moves within the tract. Whatever the etiology, however, the characteristic presenting symptoms are those of *renal colic:* agonizing, excruciating pain usually beginning in the costovertebral angle and which the patient reports as occurring suddenly and intermittently. This pain characteristically radiates along the course of the ureter—from the lumbar area of the flank, and then to the abdominal region, and finally to the groin or testis or labia of the affected side. The patient often experiences nausea and vomiting, and diaphoresis may accompany the extreme malaise.

Frequently, the patient enters the hospital as an emergency admission, and alleviation of the pain is commonly the immediate treatment that is instituted. Most patients are extremely apprehensive and will thrash about while crying out in pain. Thus it is almost impossible to begin any type of medical management until the pain is alleviated. Once the analgesic has begun to effect the relief of the acute symptom, the patient usually becomes less agitated and further treatment may be initiated. Periods of nausea and vomiting associated with renal colic often restrict fluid intake—resulting in dehydration of the individual; in such cases, the doctor will begin the IV administration of fluids. If the patient is able to take oral fluids, one of the main responsibilities of the student is the forcing of fluids. The forcing of fluids in this instance has a twofold purpose: to hydrate the patient and to flush the stone from the urinary tract. The student should also remember that—since most urinary calculi pass out of the tract spontaneously—*each voided specimen must be strained* so that passage of the stone will be detected. There are strainers made expressly for the entrapment of urinary calculi. However, when this special urinary strainer is not available, a very fine meshed gauze or muslin bedpan cover will usually serve the purpose. Ambulation also aids in the passage of stones, and—if he is not under continuous sedation for pain—the patient should be encouraged to walk about on the unit. If there are bilateral ureteral calculi, anuria (absence of urine in the bladder) may result.

A free stone in the bladder also presents a characteristic set of symptoms. Some patients complain of interruption of their urinary flow when voiding. This may be associated with pain radiating down the penile shaft, and it usually means that the stone has rolled over the bladder neck during micturition, causing an interrupted flow and pain. Frequency and urgency are often associated with these symptoms and reflect an underlying cystitis. Other patients may give a history of inability to void except in "certain positions;" the change of position serves to move the stone off the bladder neck to permit urinary outflow. The aforementioned symptoms may be associated with considerable hematuria when movement of the stone causes scraping of the wall of the bladder.

The *staghorn stone* is a large stone which *occupies and conforms to the shape of the kidney pelvis and calyces* (see Fig. 1). It is usually composed of calcium phosphate. Rarely does laboratory analysis reveal oxalate stones in staghorn form. The patient with this type of calculus complains of a dull, aching flank pain. The pain may occur only when he changes position suddenly or is jolted in some way. This type of stone is often associated with an infection in the upper tract; the nurse may observe chills and fever in the patient as well as signs of easy fatigue, loss of appetite, and generalized malaise. If this stone causes prolonged obstruction at the ureteropelvic junction, the trapped urine may result in a marked hydronephrosis; a palpable or visible mass in the flank may result. When hydronephrosis occurs, there is enlargement of the kidney pelvis and concurrent atrophy of parenchymal tissue because of the pressure of accumulated urine in the pelvis. The resultant renal damage leads to toxicity as a result of the inevitable azotemia—retention of nitrogenous wastes in the blood due to impaired renal function. Such a patient will usually manifest signs of lethargy, nausea, vomiting, or periods of disorientation.

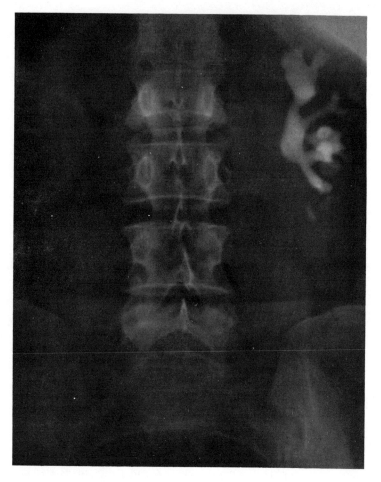

Fig. 1. A staghorn calculus is apparent in this intravenous pyelogram (IVP). (Courtesy of Department of Radiodiagnosis, St. Vincent's Hospital and Medical Center of New York.)

THE FORMATION OF CALCULI

It is seldom possible to determine the exact etiology of calculus formation, but two factors seem to be of paramount importance: the precipitation of urinary salts normally found suspended in the urine, and the presence of a nucleus for these salts to collect around. Calculi are most frequently found to be composed of urates and uric acid crystals, which make up the composition of more than half of the calculi found. The uric acid crystals precipitate out of solution in the kidney pelvis and stones form. Uric acid stones are small, hard, and yellow to reddish-brown in appearance. The acid pH of urine is favorable to their formation. Phosphates and carbonates of calcium make up the next largest group of stones found in the urinary tract. They are gray-white to yellow-white in appearance. Oxalates make up only a small percentage of the stones found; and the smooth, yellow-brown, waxy-looking cystine stones (as well as the xanthine stones) make up the smallest percentage. Various substances in the urinary tract may act as nuclei for calculus formation. Foreign bodies such as small shreds of epithelium from tissue slough, bacterial masses, red or white blood cells, or a tumor mass may become a nucleus for stone formation.

A diet deficient in vitamin A may predispose to calculus formation. Since vitamin A is concerned with the integrity of the skin and mucous membrane, its deficiency is often responsible for the shredding of the epithelium of the urinary tract. Such shreds of epithelium become foreign bodies which may act as nuclei for stone formation. Deficiency of vitamin A is also thought to be responsible for the deposit of oxalates and phosphates in the urinary tract because that vitamin is involved in the efficient functioning of the basic nutritional processes of the body.

Increased intake of vitamin D (hypervitaminosis D) potentiates an increase in the absorption of calcium from the intestine so that excretion of calcium by the kidney increases. The excessive amount of calcium salts may precipitate out of the urine, with calculus formation resulting. Individuals are also predisposed to this condition if their diets are high in cod, salmon, and other fish, as well as egg yolk and/or whole milk. When a variety of vitamin supplements are taken in addition, the incidence of calculus formation is even higher.

Urinary stasis resulting from obstruction or stagnation in the calyces may lead to stone formation. This condition causes blockage of the elimination of wastes normally excreted, so that a nucleus for calculus formation is formed. On the other hand, inadequate fluid intake usually leads to the concentration of urine. Since there is insufficient solution to keep the crystals in suspension, they precipitate out and stone formation is favored.

Infection, especially by urea-splitting organisms, also encourages the formation of calculi. The urea-splitting process causes ammonium ions to be given off, which tend to alkalinize the urine—creating an environment which favors calcium phosphate and calcium carbonate calculus formation. The student should remember that the infective organisms which travel to the stagnant urine in the urinary tract have usually come from a focus somewhere else in the body. Therefore, keeping the patient adequately hydrated and observing output in relation to intake—or maintaining a patent drainage system to effect optimum outflow of urinary drainage—is essential to the prevention of stone formation.

Metabolic diseases such as primary hyperparathyroidism and gout may also be contributory factors in calculus formation. Primary hyperparathyroidism leads to calcium metabolism imbalance which results in an increase in serum and urinary calcium. This excess calcium may crystallize out of solution and cause calculus formation. Patients on medication for the arthritis of gout may show an increase of urate crystals in their urine. The action of the medications prescribed for this disorder is to block tubular reabsorption of uric acid; this results in an increase of urate crystals in the urine. Again, precipitation of these crystals predisposes the individual to calculous disease.

The last of the factors that predispose to calculus formation is immobilization. The bedridden patient and the patient with a fracture are good candidates. They cannot move about freely, and stasis of urine in the lower calyces of the kidney —because of positional limitations—makes the urine trapped there a desirable environment for bacterial invasion. With this in mind, the importance of frequent positional changes should assume an even greater significance for the student. The hypercalciuria (increase of calcium in urine) resulting from bone demineralization during the healing process of fractures may also be a factor in the formation of urinary calculi. However, some authorities believe that increases in calciuria are negligible since the increased solubility of calcium in acid urine would allay the hazard of calculus formation.

DIAGNOSTIC PROCEDURES

The *history* given by the patient is one of the most significant contributions to the diagnosis of calculous disease. The presenting symptoms, dietary habits, health records, and family history all play an important role in ascertaining the patient's diagnosis in this particular urologic disorder. However, whether the patient is a reliable historian or not, there are many diagnostic procedures which may be utilized toward this end; some are more commonly utilized than others.

A *KUB* may be ordered for the patient presenting with signs and symptoms of calculous disease. This flat plate of the kidney, ureters, and bladder often proves helpful in locating a stone within the urinary tract. The IVP (intravenous pyelogram) is another x-ray film that is usually ordered as a means of outlining calculi within the tract (see Fig. 1). Radiopaque dye is injected intravenously and is filtered from the blood by the kidneys. As the dye is excreted into the urinary collecting system, the kidney pelves, ureters, and bladder are outlined. The stones often appear as dull, dark areas within the contrast media, or they may be seen blocking the passage of the dye in its course downward from the kidney pelvis.

Blood studies characteristically include serum calcium, phosphorus, and uric acid determinations. The doctor is most interested in increased percentage levels in the blood as this is a good indication of urinary concentrations of these elements; such information sheds light on the composition of the particular calculus under investigation.

On *urinalysis*, microscopic hematuria (related to trauma caused by stone passage) and pyuria (related to concurrent infection) may be in evidence. If the patient enters with renal colic, gross hematuria may be observed secondary to stone movement in the ureter. Urine is known to contain major end products of protein and mineral metabolism, as well as inorganic salts and pigments. The number of grams per day of each element excreted in the urine of healthy individuals falls within relative ranges. Thus, 24-hour specimens (when ordered) provide a means of measuring increases in the amount of a particular element being excreted. This aids the doctor in determining the possible composition of the calculus; 24-hour urine specimens for calcium, phosphorus, or uric acid determination (elements from which most calculi are derived) may be ordered. The student should insure that collection receptacles are clearly labeled with the patient's name, unit number, date of the collection, and the time interval during which the specimen was obtained. Collections of this kind are usually started toward the end of the night tour of duty so that completion and placement in the laboratory for analysis can be expedited with minimal delay. The nurse should consult the hospital laboratory manual for the proper method of collection (some specimens must be kept iced) because a specimen that is improperly collected will give inaccurate results. Improper collection also imposes additional expense to the patient by necessitating a repeat collection and analysis; it also makes for a longer hospitalization as well as for increased anxiety and irritability of the patient.

As a reminder to personnel on the unit and to the patient himself—if he is allowed to strain his own urine—voided specimens should be strained before being discarded. "*Strain all urine*" should be marked clearly in red on 3-inch tape and secured to the foot of the patient's bed and over the disposal unit in the utility room. If the stone is passed, care must be taken to prevent its loss as laboratory analysis will determine the composition. In this way the etiology of its formation may be ascertained. It is for this reason that all urine should be strained. Urinary calculi may be minute in dimension and, therefore, easily lost if any loosely woven mesh material is used for the purpose. When racking of urine is ordered, a means of gross examination of urine—for crystalline content, other sediment, and color—is afforded. Racking is customarily ordered if the urine is grossly bloody or contains heavy sediment, and is usually discontinued when the specimens clear. To rack a specimen, the student should *agitate each voided collection* before pouring a small amount of it into a test tube. The doctor should be notified as to where the series of specimens is being kept, and the student should summarize the findings on the chart in the nurses' notes. Specimens may usually be discarded after the doctor has seen them, or may be saved for a 24-hour period and then discarded.

The Sulkowitch test offers a quantitative method for observing increased amounts of calcium in urine. To assist in the evaluation of whether a 24-hour specimen for calculus determination is indicated, a Sulkowitch test may be ordered. The patient's calcium intake is usually restricted for three to four days prior to the test; this involves a limited-to-total restriction of milk and milk products in the diet. Then a urine specimen is obtained. When 2 ml of Sulkowitch reagent is added to 5 ml of urine, calcium precipitates out of solution. The results are determined from the speed of precipitation and the density of the cloud of calcium that forms.

Specific gravity determination is usually made at this time also; if the results of calcium precipitation are strongly positive in addition to the finding of a low specific gravity, hypercalciuria exists and a 24-hour urine collection for calcium determination is usually ordered.

Cystoscopy is seldom utilized as a diagnostic procedure for calculous disease.

METHODS OF TREATMENT AND NURSING CARE

Conservative treatment of the patient with urinary calculi basically involves elimination of the causes of the disease and supportive care during the acute phase. During the recuperative interval, teaching the patient about the causative factors of the disease and preventive measures necessary to prevent recurrence also plays an important part in the conservative treatment and care of these patients. Dietary considerations are equally important. If the patient is prone to calcium stone formation, milk and cheeses should be limited in his diet. Such a patient is usually placed on a low calcium diet. When a phosphate stone is found, a combined low calcium, moderate to low phosphorus, or an acid-ash diet may be ordered for the patient. These diets are often difficult to enforce because of the lack of variety of foods.

Episodes of calculus formation may often be traced to the patient's reverting to previous dietary habits. A urinary acidifier such as cranberry juice is frequently suggested for the phosphate stone former. Since an alkaline environment favors the formation of these stones, an approach to prevention is to insure an acid pH of the urine. Because of the untoward side effects of many urinary acidifying drugs in patients with cardiac, hepatic, and renal handicaps, and because of the distasteful flavor of others, ascorbic acid is being utilized (Murphy and Zelman, 1965). Ascorbic acid has proved effective and is palatable.

To bind phosphates in the intestine, some form of aluminum hydroxide gel may be prescribed for the phosphate stone former. For the uric acid or cystine stone former, the low purine or alkaline-ash diet is indicated. The student is encouraged to consult the diet manual regarding these diets during the course of clinical experiences so as to be familiar with the foods which comprise them. And nurses should *always* check to insure that the patient has been given a copy of the prescribed diet *before* discharge. In many institutions the nutritionist or head dietician is sent a diet slip and automatically visits and instructs the patient regarding the diet. However, the nurse should make sure that this has been done before the patient is discharged because it is an extremely important aspect of his care. All of these patients should be encouraged to maintain a good fluid intake. Most of them presenting with urinary calculi may be managed adequately on a dietary regimen. However, for a small percentage of patients, more rigorous intervention is indicated.

Although most calculi are small enough to pass out of the tract spontaneously, a few are too large to accomplish this and surgical removal (called a lithotomy) is necessary. When a stone is to be removed through the *parenchyma* of the kidney (nephrolithotomy), through or from the *pelvis* of the kidney (pyelolithotomy), or from the upper two-thirds of the *ureter* (ureterolithotomy), an incision is made in the flank (between the ribs and hip). This is often a generous incision that extends from the area of the costovertebral angle to within 2 or 3 inches below the level of the nipple on the chest wall of the affected side. Whenever an operation is performed in this area, there are specific responsibilities indicated for the nurse. One of them is to *insure the adequate ventilation* of the patient since the location and extent of the incision make the prevention of atelectasis a distinct management problem. If the student will place both palms on either side of the rib cage and take a deep breath—being sure to note the anatomic involvement necessary for the execution of this act—it will become more understandable why the patient with a flank incision of this nature would experience great pain when taking deep breaths postoperatively. Such a patient will often tend to shallow-breathe and shallow-cough, their efforts often resembling throat-clearing activity. Thus adequate medication for pain is essential—especially in the first 48 hours following surgical intervention—if the patient is to be expected to cough and/or deep-breathe. The nurse should be sure to medicate the patient as ordered before initiating treatments. The patient must work to clear his lungs during the early postoperative period, and although rest is also of importance the student should not consider medication for pain as being given solely for the comfort of the patient. It is also the means through which he will be enabled to turn, cough, and breathe deeply. He must be encouraged to *make positional changes* at least every 2 hours unless specifically ordered otherwise by the doctor. The turning may include the operative side if the patient can tolerate it. Maximum cooperation is usually obtained when the patient is permitted to turn himself. A pillow positioned along his back will give additional support as well as encouragement to remain as positioned until the next change. Giving mechanical support (splinting) to the back and chest by utilizing a towel, half sheet, or scultetus binder with tails held firmly in the hands of the nurse will make coughing a less traumatic experience. Such support will also encourage the patient to expand the lungs fully when taking deep breaths. If a nephrostomy tube is in place, the patient may be tilted slightly toward that side and propped with pillows for support. The tubing should be checked for kinks and tension (or pulling); these are to be guarded against.

Special mention must be given to the *care of the nephrostomy tube* (or ureterostomy tube) if one is present. Often, if a large stone is removed, tissue irritation and edema will cause a narrowing of the lumen at the UP junction or within the ureter. An indwelling catheter is therefore indicated to temporarily divert the urinary flow. This catheter is seldom a self-retaining catheter, and is thus held in place by a skin suture or an adhesive tab taped to the skin at the incisional site. A drainage system (usually a gravity drainage system) is attached to the indwelling catheter, and care must be taken to guard against twisting or kinking of the catheter and drainage tubing. This would lead to obstruction to the outflow of urine and predispose the patient to stasis and infection in the upper urinary tract. Such infection can lead to serious renal damage. To prevent this, the nurse should best secure the tubing to the skin with an adhesive tape at (or immediately above) the level of the anterior iliac crest of the pelvis on the affected side. This will insure against tension or twisting of the tubing whether the patient is in bed or ambulating. After a few days, the catheter is usually removed by the doctor, and the necessity for frequent dressing changes should be anticipated. There may be large amounts of drainage present even if an indwelling catheter has been used as there will be extravasation (escape of fluid into the surrounding tissue) of urine around the tissue drain or drainage tube. When the nurse makes entries on the chart, the drainage on the dressing may thus be described as urosanguinous if blood-tinged, or urinary if clear.

Observation for hemorrhage, especially following nephrolithotomy or pyelolithotomy, is also of great importance. The kidney parenchyma is highly vascular, and any surgical interruption of its tissue carries a high risk for hemorrhage in the postoperative period. It must be remembered that the patient should be turned slightly when dressing observations are being made; this will permit a view of the *back* of the dressing, as drainage will flow toward the back of the dressing and may not be visible on superficial examination. The *amount* (moderate, small, scant, etc.) and *color* (sanguinous, urosanguinous, amber, etc.) of the drainage should be recorded in the nurses' notes and communicated to the other members of the nursing team during report time.

The nurse must also be aware that *observation for distention* is another of the priority needs of the patient with a flank incision. These patients usually begin intake of oral fluids on the first postoperative day. Thereafter, the nurses on the unit will have the responsibility of forcing fluids. Since distention seems to be a postoperative problem with these patients—abdominal distention resulting from paralytic ileus of reflex origin —*warm fluids* should be given initially. The nurse should also make frequent observations of the patient's abdomen, or inquire about the passage of flatus and/or borborygmus (rumbling in the bowels); and these observations should also be included in the nurses' notes (examples: *no abdominal distention noted; abdomen firmly [or softly] distended; passing flatus frequently [or occasionally]*, etc.). Oral fluids are usually started slowly and the nurse must observe for signs of distention. In some cases the patient is kept NPO for 24 to 48 hours and may return to the unit with a gastric tube in place. These are prophylactic measures; however, if distention occurs in spite of the usual precautionary or prophylactic measures, the patient may usually be given a rectal tube. Prostigmine injections with a rectal tube being given 20 minutes after the injection and/or carminative (gas-expelling) enemas may also be ordered to remedy the condition by encouraging peristalsis of the bowel.

Renal and perirenal abscess formation is usually treated by incision and drainage of the abscess. Since the incision is in the same area as that made for the excision of calculi from the kidney or kidney pelvis, the key aspects of nursing care previously mentioned apply in this instance also. However, regarding the postoperative course of the patient, hemorrhage is most likely to occur either in the immediate postoperative period or on the eighth through twelfth postoperative days— the period when tissue sloughing usually occurs in healing. For this reason, the patient who has been ambulatory since the second or third postoperative day may be ordered on bed rest for a short interval of time. The nurse should allay fears in these instances by explaining that this is merely a precautionary measure and not an indication of a negative change in condition.

When a calculus is removed from the lower third of the ureter or from the bladder (a cystolithotomy), the incision is made suprapubically and the care is similar to that discussed for the suprapubic prostatectomy patient (see Chapter 6). Many times a bladder stone may be too large to pass out of the urinary tract through the urethra, but may not be large enough to warrant a suprapubic approach into the bladder. Such a calculus may be *crushed* (litholapaxy) with a stone crusher (lithotrite) that is passed transurethrally (see Fig. 2) in much the same manner as the cystoscope is passed. Preoperatively, *continuous* bladder irrigations with an acid solution

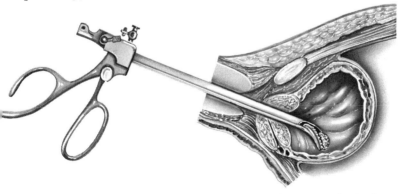

Fig. 2. A lithotrite. Note the grippers which may hold a stone prior to the crushing procedure. (From Roen. Atlas of Urologic Surgery. 1967. Courtesy of Appleton-Century-Crofts.)

may be ordered in an attempt to soften the stone and alter the pH of the alkaline urine which favored its formation. Phosphoric acid in strengths of 1:10,000 or 1:15,000, or urologic solution G (a solution of citric acid, sodium carbonate, and magnesium oxide) are frequently used for this purpose. Postoperatively, *intermittent* bladder irrigations may be ordered to flush out the remaining particles of the stone—sandlike sediment. Nursing care is similar to that given the patient with a transurethral prostatectomy (see Chapter 6).

A NURSING-CARE STUDY

Mr. B. is a 63-year-old man who entered the hospital with the chief complaint of left flank pain. This was his third hospital admission.

His first hospitalization had occurred 11 years prior to his current admission. At that time, he was diagnosed as having a calculus in the right ureter, with pyelonephritis of the right kidney. Conservative treatment—the administration of antibiotics and the forcing of fluids—was instituted, and the symptoms subsided.

Mr. B. remained asymptomatic until 6 years thereafter, when he entered the hospital again; this time he had left flank pain. During this second hospitalization, an intravenous pyelogram (IVP) revealed a stone in the inferior calyx of the left kidney. The symptoms subsided spontaneously during this episode and the patient was discharged.

Five years later (the current admission), Mr. B. entered the hospital again. For 6 hours prior to his admission, Mr. B. has experienced left flank pain which radiated to the anterior abdominal wall. He had also experienced dysuria, frequency, and urgency —symptoms which he had not experienced during previous episodes. Hematuria was not noted when he voided; he was afebrile, and had no complaints of nausea. Mr. B. had a history of mild diabetes which was controlled by dietary measures. The tentative diagnosis on admission was left renal calculus.

Doctor's Orders—Day of Admission

1,800 caloric diabetic diet
Routine blood work
Chest x-ray
KUB, schedule for IVP
Rack and strain all urine
VSq shift
Bedrest with BRP
Urinalysis and urine for C&S
AC urines
Demerol for pain, 100 mg q. 4 h, PRN

The student familiarized the patient with the facilities available on the unit—including the bedside call system for nursing aid and the bathroom emergency call system. Then, after setting up an area in the bathroom for a rack of test tubes and a urinary strainer, the patient was told how to strain and rack his urine after voiding, the student reassuring him that his first endeavor would be supervised. Appropriate adhesive tape signs reading *"Strain all urine"* were placed conspicuously on the bed and in the bathroom by the hopper. Thereafter, the patient's vital signs were taken with special attention given to the *temperature*, since fever would make an associated infection suspect. The limitations of his physical activity were explained to the patient, and, after he was properly cleansed, a midstream urine specimen was collected and immediately sent to the laboratory for culture and sensitivity studies. A second specimen was collected and sent to the laboratory for routine urinalysis, and the AC urine schedule was begun—urine specimens being collected and tested for sugar content and acetone with the results recorded on the appropriate sheet in the patient's chart. During the course of this assignment, the student also medicated the patient as needed after she obtained a verbal description of the *site* and *quality* of the pain. The student did not assume that the patient was having pain in the same site and of the same intensity each time, for it was remembered that—as the stone travels—the site and quality of the pain may vary at any given time.

The nurse's notes at the end of the assignment included the patient's temperature, the color and kind of sediment present in the urine, the results of the AC urines, whether the stone had been passed, and the number of times the patient was medicated for pain. The site and quality or intensity of the pain were also noted, as well as whether the medication given was effective or not. (A recorded and reported profile of these facts helped to give the rest of the nursing team a comprehensive picture of the patient's status.)

The blood work was done and revealed a BUN (blood urea nitrogen) level of 15 mg percent—which was within the normal limits of 10 to 20 mg percent. In the evening of the second day after admission, the patient was prepared for the IVP. A cathartic was given, the patient was told that he should take nothing by mouth after midnight, and permission was obtained. The patient asked if he would be given cleansing enemas also. It was explained that no enemas would be given; in many patients the bowel becomes filled with gas following the enemas. (Gas in the bowel tends to obstruct visualization of the urinary tract.) It was further explained that the dye injected would circulate in a more concentrated form if the fluid intake was limited. The IVP revealed a ptosed left kidney enlarged in size and curvature of the left ureter.

On the fifth day after his admission, Mr. B. was premedicated for cystoscopy, and the student was careful to pull up the side rails of the bed to insure the protection of the patient while he was waiting to be taken to the cystoscopy room. Permission had been obtained the evening before, and the patient had been NPO after midnight. Cystoscopy revealed an unremarkable bladder, but retrograde

films* confirmed the IVP findings of curvature of the
left ureter with ptosed kidney. In addition, an opacity
in the parenchyma adjacent to the lower calyx was
revealed. When the patient was returned to the unit
he was kept on bedrest and given pain medication
as needed for the discomfort he felt subsequent to the
passage of the cystoscope. His vital signs were taken
periodically with special attention being given to his
temperature; any significant change suggests the possibility of infection secondary to instrumentation.
Mr. B. was also encouraged to force fluids in order
to compensate for the long interval during which
fluids had been withheld. The student was careful to
note and record the time, amount, and color of the
first voiding since *anuria* and/or *hematuria* secondary to instrumentation of the urinary tract may occur
after cystoscopic examination. (Complaints of chills
should also alert the nurse to the possibility of infection; in addition to providing more warm covering, the patient's temperature should be taken.)

Since the retrograde films had confirmed the
distortion in the parenchyma noted on IVP, it was
necessary for the doctors to rule out the possibility
of a tumor mass within the parenchyma. A renal
arteriogram (x-ray of the circulation to the kidney
and kidney parenchyma) was therefore ordered on
the evening of the sixth day of Mr. B.'s hospitalization. The inquinal region was then shaved bilaterally
in preparation for the eventual introduction of a
catheter (via femoral puncture) into the femoral
artery during the arteriogram procedure. Mr. B.

---

* Retrograde pyelography is accomplished when radiopaque dye is injected into the renal pelvis via *ureteral* catheters which have been
threaded through the cystocope (see Fig. 4, Chap. 3). The *working lens*
of the cystoscope accommodates the two catheters which are threaded into
the bladder, through the ureteral orifices, up the ureters, and into the
kidney pelvis. Radiopaque dye may then be injected into the lumen of
the ureteral catheters through their external tip, and in this manner
the dye may be delivered to the renal pelvis. The injected dye is forced
upward, fills the pelvis, travels down the ureters by peristalsis and
enters the bladder. X-rays are taken from the time that dye enters the
pelvis, and the dye is expelled from the tract when the patient voids.

was allowed fluids until 6 o'clock the next morning, but they were withheld thereafter.

On the morning of the seventh day after the patient's admission, a student premedicated him as ordered and—after pulling up the siderails on the bed—checked the chart to make sure that all of the latest blood studies had been attached. Then the patient was sent to the x-ray department for the renal arteriogram. Upon his return to the unit, his vital signs were taken over a 4-hour period—four times at 30-minute intervals, and twice at hourly intervals—so that any untoward effect on the circulatory system could be noted and reported. The student observed the left inguinal area of the puncture site for bleeding or hematoma by *lifting* the pressure dressing periodically. (If a hematoma seems to be enlarging the blood oozing from the vessel at the puncture site may often be stopped by the application of firm pressure from the nurse's fingers positioned on the bandage, over the puncture site. If the enlargement continues thereafter, the doctor should be notified immediately.) An ice cap was applied to the left groin for a 4-hour period also, and this was removed periodically to prevent ice burns to the skin. Mr. B. remained on bedrest for the rest of that day. The arteriogram revealed a normal vascular supply to the kidney, and an intrarenal stone in the lower pole of the left kidney was demonstrated.

By the eighth day after admission, the work-up on Mr. B. had been completed and preoperative nephrolithotomy orders were written.* The patient had been moderately apprehensive throughout the diagnostic work-up period, and it seemed very difficult to allay his fears. When this aspect of his care was discussed early in the course of his hospitaliza-

---

* A *lithotomy* is the removal of a stone. The prefix attached to the word stem refers to the place or cavity from which the stone is being removed. Thus a *nephro*lithotomy is the removal of a stone from the parenchyma of the kidney; a *pyelo*lithotomy, the removal of a stone from the kidney pelvis; a *uretero*lithotomy, the removal of a stone from the ureter; and a *cysto*lithotomy, the removal of a stone from the bladder.

tion at one of the nursing-care conferences, the team members who had taken care of the patient communicated individual approaches to the resolution of this problem. After lengthy discussion, the concensus was that the purpose of all treatments should be carefully explained to Mr. B. by the team leader in simple terms far enough in advance of the treatment to allow him to accept its purpose and necessity and, consequently, to cooperate with the staff. A positive, gentle, but firm approach to the implementation of nursing care was to be adopted; it was also decided that various members of the nursing team should stop at Mr. B.'s bedside periodically for brief chats to show their interest in his well-being and to afford him an opportunity to express his thoughts. The problem-solving approach to Mr. B.'s emotional needs proved successful because *consistency* was introduced into his new environment. He often remarked that he had confidence in the staff; but each new procedure filled him with fears about his physical condition, and these fears were manifested by his demanding—almost argumentative—behavior. If authoritarian or reprehensive techniques had been employed by the various members of the nursing team, time would have been wasted and the patient's anxiety and hostility levels would have increased. As things worked out, however, the approach implemented by the nursing team helped the patient to cope with his apprehension and to cooperate with the staff.

The necessity for positional changes, coughing, and deep-breathing activities in the postoperative period was explained to Mr. B. and, on the ninth day after admission, the patient was taken to the operating room for a nephrolithotomy of the left kidney. When he returned to the unit, the student who had been assigned to his care took his vital signs, observed the dressing over the operative site for drainage (turning the patient slightly to the right so as to obtain a view of the back of the dressing), and checked the IV equipment to be sure it was running well. Then the postoperative orders and the operative note were reviewed.

The Postoperative Orders

Vital signs q ½ h till stable, then q 1 h × 8, then q 2 h
Keep 3 units whole blood on reserve
Blood work in A.M.
NPO until passing flatus
IV fluids
Strict intake and output
Bedrest—may stand to void, OOB in chair in A.M.
Test Urine–QID—Coverage

> $1^+ =$ 5 units regular insulin
> $2^+ = 10$ units regular insulin
> $3^+ = 15$ units regular insulin
> $4^+ = 20$ units regular insulin
> If negative = no insulin

Nembutal 100 mg q h.s., PRN
Demerol 100 mg q 4 h, PRN for pain

The pyelostomy tube (catheter in the kidney pelvis) protruding from the dressing was attached to a straight gravity drainage system, the tubing being taped to the patient's side with an adhesive tab to prevent tension, pulling, or twisting. Then the student placed a vital signs sheet, and an intake and output sheet on the patient's over-the-bed table along with the next bottle of IV solution which was to follow the one currently running in so that all would be in readiness. A mouth care set-up was placed on the bedside table and mouth care was given. A few clean combines were also placed at the bedside table so that they would be handy should the dressing need reinforcement. A box of tissues was taped to the bed with a strip of adhesive so as to be within reach but stationary, and a paper bag for tissue disposal was pinned to the side of the bed.

The vital signs were taken as ordered thereafter, and the patient was encouraged to deep-breathe and cough every 2 hours. The nurse encouraged the patient to place his right hand over the operative site

to lend support during the intervals of deep-breathing and coughing. The nurse's hands were placed
beside the patient's to lend additional support at
these times; immediately after those ventilation activities were completed, the patient's position was
changed. The time taken to implement each treatment was kept to a minimum, and Mr. B. was
allowed to rest between treatments.

The student realized that the kidney is a highly
vascular organ, and was especially alert to observing
the dressing for sanguinous drainage. The operative
note had revealed that—in addition to the pyelostomy
tube—the patient had two penrose drains in the incision. The dressing remained dry, however, and
*uro*sanguinous fluid was draining through the pyelostomy tube. Urine tests were done as ordered, and
the student was prepared to notify the team leader
if the acetone test became positive. Six hours after
the patient was returned to the unit, he was assisted
to a standing position by two team members and
voided 90 ml of blood-tinged urine. The student kept
an accurate record of the output—voided and via
pyelostomy tube—and of the IV intake, totaling both
when the day's assignment had been completed.

The patient remained drowsy most of the time,
but when he was awake he was reassured that the
operation had been successful. The nurse was patient
while encouraging Mr. B. to take deep breaths and
to cough, and he was praised when he accomplished
the task—whether the effort was productive of mucus
or not. Diaphoresis was noted after these exertional
episodes and after injections of pain-medication had
been given. Gown changes were made accordingly,
and Mr. B. was reassured that the episodes of
diaphoresis were to be expected.

After the morning bath had been given on the
first postoperative day, the patient was assisted out
of bed and into a chair which had been placed by the
bedside. He tolerated this activity well, and completed his oral hygiene while in the sitting position.
Medication had been given before the bath was

started so that it would take effect by the time the patient was to be assisted out of bed; this made the activity easier for Mr. B. to accomplish. However, the student remained with the patient during the interval that he was up and out of bed to insure his safety. His vital signs had stabilized the day before, so he had been placed on 4-hour observations. When he went back to bed, his pulse and blood pressure were taken and then the stethoscope was positioned on the abdominal wall. Bowel sounds were audible. During morning rounds, although IV fluid orders were written, the patient was allowed ice chips by mouth, being restricted to no more than 15 ml per hour. The nurse put a cup containing what was approximated to be a 4-hour supply of ice chips at the bedside, and the patient was warned to put only a small amount in his mouth at any given time. The dressing remained dry and the drainage from the pyelostomy tube continued to be urosanguinous. He continued to void in small amounts. Antibiotic therapy was started, and it was explained that this was a precautionary measure frequently instituted after surgical procedures.

Mr. B. balked when he was asked to cough and deep-breathe, and, even though he had been medicated, he complained of soreness in the shoulder and lower-back regions of the affected side. It was explained that his position on the operating table was the probable cause of the associated soreness; hyperextension of the left side had been necessary for maximum visualization during the operation. To give additional support to the operative area during the periods of coughing, a half sheet was placed around the area and held securely at the sternum by the nursing student. This seemed to make the coughing easier, although it was unproductive. At other times when Mr. B. hesitated to cough, he explained that he was afraid he would burst his stitches. The student reassured him that the stitches had been securely placed and that with support given during the coughing activity such an occurrence would be almost impossible.

By the second postoperative day, the bowel sounds were more active, and warm, clear liquids were allowed although IV fluids were continued. The patient was allowed to ambulate progressively thereafter; he was instructed to remember to keep the gravity drainage receptacle attached by tubing to the pyelostomy tube at arm's length and always well below the level of the dressing when he was walking about or sitting up. His coughing was productive, and support was given with the half sheet periodically to encourage really deep breathing and vigorous coughing. Since the patient was passing flatus by the third postoperative day, a full fluid diet was allowed and intake of liquids was encouraged. Intravenous fluids were discontinued. Mr. B. was voiding in moderate amounts even though about 25 percent of the total urinary output was draining through the pyelostomy tube.

On the fourth postoperative day the urine was still blood-tinged and the patient was found to have a temperature of 101 degrees. The student assigned to his care assessed his priority need as being fluid intake since his total output had diminished and his fluid intake had not exceeded 2,100 ml on the preceding day. The patient's preference for liquid refreshment was ascertained and those fluids chosen were alternately urged. The elevation resolved itself uneventfully.

On the fifth postoperative day Mr. B. was allowed a regular low calcium diet; the following day, the dressing and alternate sutures were removed by the doctor. An order was written giving the nurses permission to change the dressing PRN thereafter. The vital signs were taken once each day at this juncture. The patient remained afebrile from the fifth through the seventh postoperative day, so the antibiotics were discontinued. A urinary-tract antiseptic was ordered because the pyelostomy tube was still in place, and the AC urine tests were discontinued because the results had been consistently negative. The daily blood work—the hematocrit being of special concern to the doctor—was advanced to triweekly reports; the patient's vital signs remained stable. The pyelostomy tube was withdrawn from the pelvis of the kidney but was left in the tract; on the eighth postoperative day it was completely removed. The remaining sutures were removed also. Mr. B.'s mood became elevated and he enjoyed visiting with other patients more and with the staff less.

When the drains were withdrawn 1½ inches on the tenth postoperative day, a small amount of serous drainage was noted; the dressing was changed as needed. By the twelfth postoperative day, however, the drains were removed and only scant amounts of drainage were observed from the operative site thereafter until the area was completely healed. The patient was scheduled for IVP with post-voiding cystogram (x-ray of the bladder after the patient has voided following an IVP). The report of the IVP was received about three days later; the tract was patent. Mr. B. was elated about the report and the course of his progress. The blood work was cut, and the charting of intake and output was discontinued. The nutritionist came to the unit to discuss the low calcium diet with the patient and left a printed outline of the diet with him. After her departure, Mr. B. questioned one of the nurses about the limitations of the diet and its relationship to his stone-forming tendency. He seemed to understand the reason for the restriction and promised to follow the diet when he went home. He was discharged the next day.

REFERENCES

1. Cooper, E. M. Renal colic. Penn. Med., 69:49–51, 1966.
2. Editorial. Urinary calculi. J. Florida Med. Ass., 53:128–132, 1966.
3. Elliot, J. S. Urinary calculus disease. Surg. Clin. N. Amer. 45:1393–1404, 1965.
4. Gershoff, S. N. The formation of urinary stones. Metabolism 13:875–887, 1964.

5. King., J. S., Jr. Etiologic factors involved in urolithiasis: A review of recent research. J. Urol., 97:583–591, 1967.
6. Martin, F. J. A critical evaluation of the Sulkowitch test for urine calcium. Med. J. Aust., 1:936–938, 1966.
7. Mayer, G. G., et al. Metabolic studies on the formation of calcium oxalate stones, with special emphasis on Vitamin B_6 and uric acid metabolism. Bull. N.Y. Acad. Med., 44:28–44, 1968.
8. Mulvaney, W. P. Prevention of calcification of in-dwelling catheters. Arch. Phys. Med., 45:610–613, 1964.
9. Murphy, F. J., and Zelman, S. Ascorbic acid as a urinary acidifying agent. J. Urol., 94:297–303, 1965.
10. Nordin, B. E. C., and Hodgkinson, A. Urolithiasis. Advances Intern. Med., 13:155–182, 1967.
11. Roen, P. R. Atlas of Urologic Surgery. New York, Appleton-Century-Crofts, 1967.
12. Schroeder, L. M. The hazards of immobility: Effects on urinary function. Amer. J. Nurs., 67:790–792, 1967.
13. Urological Symposium: The Recurring Urinary Calculus. J. Florida Med. Ass., 53:115–120, 1966.
14. Vermeulen, C. W., et al. On the nature of the stone-forming process. J. Urol., 94:176–186, 1965.

6

Characteristics and Care
of the Patient with
Benign Prostatic Hypertrophy

Benign prostatic hypertrophy is the terminology used to describe hyperplasia of adenomatous tissue within the prostate gland. The periurethral tissue (tissue surrounding the prostatic urethra) of the gland undergoes nonmalignant, nodular enlargement which compresses the remaining normal tissue laterally toward the outer capsule. It should be remembered that the prostatic portion of the urethra and the bladder neck enclose the innermost aspect of the prostate while the rest of the gland is surrounded by a dense capsule.

As the periurethral tissue enlarges, it extends upward into the bladder to form a pouch or recess that traps urine and prevents complete emptying during micturition (see Fig. 1). This incomplete emptying leads to increased amounts of residual urine's being retained in the bladder. In addition to the upward extension, the hyperplastic tissue moves *inwardly*, encroaching on the walls of the prostatic urethra and on the bladder neck. This early stage of hypertrophy causes a narrowing of the urinary outlet, and a man over 50 (such en-

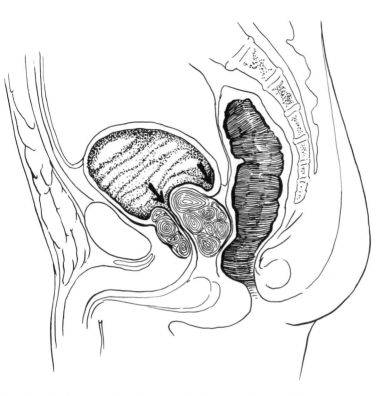

Fig. 1. The dynamics of benign prostatic hypertrophy. Note the recess within the bladder behind the hypertrophied gland; this retains urine during micturition. Also note how the hypertrophied gland causes a narrowing at the bladder neck and urethral outlet.

largement usually begins after the fifth decade of life) may start having symptoms of dysuria and frequency. Characteristic local symptoms are: difficulty in starting the urinary stream, difficulty in maintaining the stream, diminished caliber and force of the stream, and "dribbling" of urine after micturition has been completed. *Nocturia* is the best index of frequency; a man may report that his rest is interrupted from four to eight times during the night because of the need to void. The residual urine in the bladder may increase from between 30 to 100 ml to 200 to 300 ml or more; the resulting stagnation predisposes the individual to cystitis. It is not unusual, therefore, to hear complaints of urgency and "burning" on urination as the disease process progresses.

While obstruction to urinary outflow gradually increases, the bladder musculature endeavors to compensate for the increased urinary residual and for the increased intravesical pressure. Atonicity often results. An analogy between the bladder and a balloon seems appropriate at this juncture. Before it is inflated, a balloon has tone, turgor, and a well-defined contour. However, after it has been inflated and the gas has been allowed to escape, the observer will note that the walls of the balloon appear wrinkled and the contour is distorted. Atonicity results from the forced stretching of the walls of the balloon. Much the same process occurs with the bladder musculature when there is obstruction at the bladder neck. The detrusor muscle overworks in an effort to overcome the resistance at the bladder neck, and it becomes hypertrophied. The sagging bands of atonic, hypertrophied muscle form *trabeculations* which appear as trellised structures protruding from the bladder wall. The trabeculations represent bladder decompensation and may be visualized during cystoscopy.

The increased intravesical pressure and the compromised integrity of the detrusor muscle often lead to relaxation of the normal control at the ureteral orifice.

The same degree of bilateral involvement of the upper urinary tract seldom occurs, but the gradual dilatation of a ureter and kidney pelvis is referred to as *hydroureter* and *hydronephrosis*, respectively (see Fig. 2). As the capacity of the kidney pelvis increases, the urine retained may exert enough pressure to cause atrophy of the renal parenchyma. If the obstruction is not relieved, pressure above the obstruction persists—backing up to the level of the kidney—and impaired renal function will result. When complete obstruction

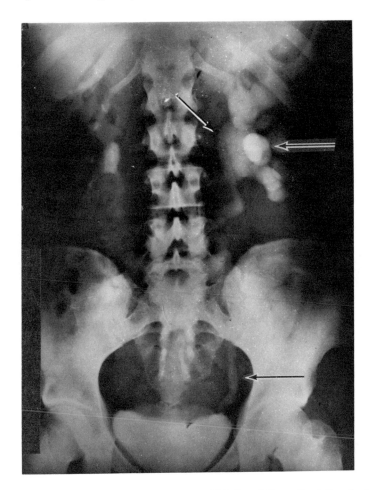

Fig. 2. The IVP. This view shows enormous dilatation of the entire left collecting system. Hydroureter and hydronephrosis are clearly discernible. (Courtesy of Department of Radiodiagnosis, St. Vincent's Hospital and Medical Center of New York.)

occurs and the individual is unable to void, he is said to be in *retention*.

Pain is not characteristic of the patient who presents with benign prostatic hypertrophy, but it may exist if a calculus (or calculi) has developed in the bladder secondary to the obstructive process, if a severe infection (e.g., cystitis or cysto-prostatitis) is present, or if the patient is experiencing acute retention. An individual who has been complaining of minor or moderate symptoms suddenly cannot void and experiences cramplike pain in the lower abdominal region. The pain may radiate to the glans penis, to the perineum, and/or to the lumbar region. *Acute retention* is the terminology given to such a sudden onset of retention. *Chronic retention*, however, results from a gradual increase of residual urine which distends the bladder with enormous amounts of urine. The individual discovers that he cannot void, but experiences dribbling of urine at irregular intervals instead. This is often overflow incontinence. Pain is absent in this process because the sensory receptors of the bladder have atrophied from the continuous, high intravesical pressure and they do not function. It is this long-standing type of retention that predisposes the individual to severe complications of obstruction that have been mentioned.

Generalized symptoms are usually manifested if renal function is impaired secondary to back pressure from obstruction of the lower tract; the condition represents varying degrees of uremia. Often the individual adapts to the subtle progress of impaired renal function, and symptoms such as anorexia, weight loss, dyspepsia, and irritability cause no alarm. Although the individual may be lethargic during the day and demonstrate an inability to concentrate, there may be complaints of inability to sleep during the night. Marked skin irritation, constipation, and increased thirst with a dry, coated tongue may be representative of ever-increasing renal insufficiency. Table 1 outlines the signs and symptoms of benign prostatic hypertrophy.

The etiology of benign prostatic hypertrophy is still a matter for conjecture. It is known that testosterone stimulates prostatic growth whereas castration causes involution of the

Table 1
BENIGN PROSTATIC HYPERTROPHY

SUMMARY OF SIGNS AND SYMPTOMS

Anatomic Changes	Symptomatology
1. As the prostate gland enlarges, it extends upward into the bladder and simultaneously constricts the prostatic urethra.	The patient complains of: a) difficulty in starting the urinary stream, b) diminished caliber of the stream, and c) diminished force of the stream. Collectively, these complaints are called symptoms of *prostatism*.
2. The hyperplastic tissue forms a pouch within the bladder which retains urine. (Behind the enlarging tissue a recess is formed within the bladder. The bladder does not empty completely during micturition because some of the urine gets trapped within the recess. Thus the amount of residual urine increases.)	The patient complains of: a) frequency, b) nocturia, and c) urgency.
3. This rising residual predisposes the patient to infection—*cystitis*.	The patient may complain of experiencing a "burning" sensation when he urinates.
4. Gradually, the enlargement produces obstruction to the outflow of urine because the bladder neck is constricted. A suprapubic bulge may be noted.	a) The patient is unable to void and has *retention* of urine. b) The patient may complain of mild to severe discomfort, depending on the amount of urine being retained in the bladder.

SOME COMPLICATIONS ARISING FROM SECONDARY OBSTRUCTION OF THE LOWER URINARY TRACT

Condition	Associated Conditions
1. Bladder decompensation.	*Trabeculations* (sagging of atonic mucous membrane between over-

Table 1 (cont.)

	worked hypertrophied muscle bands of the bladder) are representative of bladder decompensation. The stretching of the bladder musculature to accommodate the increased amounts of urine is responsible for this phenomenon.
2. Hydroureter and hydronephrosis.	The gradual dilatation of the ureters and kidney pelves as the result of obstruction to the outflow of urine leads to hydroureter and hydronephrosis. Reflux of urine in the ureters is also contributory.
3. Infection within the urinary tract.	Cystitis, ureteritis, pyelitis, etc., may occur secondary to the stasis of urine.
4. Impaired renal function.	Compression and subsequent destruction of the renal parenchyma secondary to hydronephrosis leads to impaired renal function.

gland. In animals, prostatic hyperplasia resulting from injections of estrogen has been demonstrated and subsequent testosterone injections countered the hyperplasia. Therefore, since estrogen is excreted in the urine of the male and can be isolated from testicular tissue, most authorities believe that imbalance in the normal androgen-estrogen ratio imposed by the aging process predisposes an individual to benign prostatic hypertrophy.

An individual may seek medical advice at any stage of prostatic hypertrophy. The degree of enlargement may be approximated during the rectal examination when an estimate of the amount of protrusion into the bladder can be ascertained. One plus (1+) usually refers to minimal hyperplasia and four plus (4+) to an extremely enlarged gland; two and three plus (2+, 3+) are the usual designations for varying stages intermediate between minimal and extreme hyperplasia. The symptoms and amount of distress experienced by the individual tend to vary with the degree of hypertrophy. A number of patients will consult a doctor when they notice the slightest change in urinary habits and are experiencing early symptoms of prostatism. However, others will wait until the process has progressed to the stage where they are in acute distress from retention before they seek medical advice. Fortunately, only about one-fifth of all presenting patients require surgical intervention for the relief of symptoms. If the patient enters the hospital with complaints of early symptoms of prostatism, the diagnostic work-up usually begins immediately; but if the patient enters with urinary retention, relief of that condition takes priority over other considerations.

THE DIAGNOSTIC WORK-UP

For the patient entering with early symptoms of prostatism—hesitancy in initiating the stream, diminished caliber and force of the stream, difficulty in maintaining the stream, and nocturnal frequency—a *rectal examination* and a *residual urine determination* are essential for an evaluation of the need for intervention. The rectal examination (see Fig. 3) is done to palpate the gland (the proximity of the prostate gland to the rectum should be recalled), and is accomplished by digital palpation through the rectal wall. The one-to-four-plus (1+, 2+, 3+, 4+) estimates of the degree of hypertrophy are usually made after such an examination is done. The amount of residual urine present in the bladder may be determined by either a postvoiding catheterization or by postvoiding x-rays following intravenous or retrograde pyelography. If 75 ml or more urine remains in the bladder after the patient has voided, early bladder decompensation becomes suspect and an environment conducive to bacterial invasion has been created. For accuracy, the patient should be catheterized (or x-rayed) immediately after he has voided. At times, when there is no

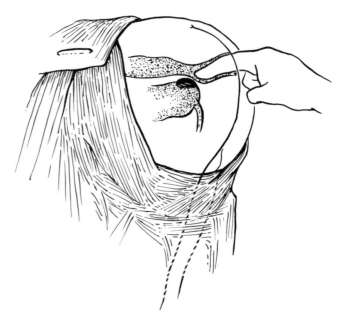

Fig. 3. The rectal examination. The proximity of the rectum to the prostate gland should be noted. **The proper draping of the patient is an essential nursing responsibility.**

orderly on the unit, the physician has to be notified and will have to come to the unit from another part of the hospital. The patient should, therefore, be instructed to notify the student *immediately after* voiding so that the doctor may be summoned to the unit. This allows only a minimum of time to pass between the patient's voiding and catheterization for residual urine determination.

The intravenous pyelogram (IVP) is a renal-function test which outlines the kidney pelves, ureters, and bladder. Since the intravenous injection of radiopaque dye accomplishes the test, the patient must sign a consent form. The dye circulates in the bloodstream, reaches the kidneys (where it is filtered from the blood), and is excreted into the urinary collecting system—outlining it while being swept downward through the tract. Thus impaired renal function (determined by the time taken for the kidneys to begin excreting the dye) may be evaluated, and complications such as hydronephrosis and hydroureter may be visualized. If films are taken while the patient is voiding (a *voiding cystogram*), the degree of bladder neck and urethral compression may be estimated by comparison of the relative diameters of the proximal and distal portions of the urethra. Urethrograms (x-ray pictures of the urethra) may also permit such visualization. Opacity in the bladder filmed after the patient has voided will reveal the amount of residual urine present.

Specific preparation of the patient may vary from institution to institution; however, the bowel is usually evacuated through the action of a cathartic, an enema, or both so that shadows from gas and feces contained in the bowel do not interfere with visualization of the urinary tract. (At this point the student should recall that the kidneys are situated retroperitoneally.) Fluid intake is usually restricted for some designated period of time prior to injection of the dye so that—with the state of dehydration thus created—it will circulate with the blood and reach the kidneys in a more concentrated form. Food is also restricted. The student should explain all this to the patient so as to elicit his cooperation. While the patient is being prepared, the student should ascertain whether he has a history of allergy or serious kidney damage as the treatment is often contraindicated in these instances. Serious reactions may occur from use of the dye in individuals who are hypersensitive. Since the dye must be filtered from the blood by the parenchymal tissue, preexisting renal damage would leave only a limited number of functional units to carry out the work.

If the student is present when the x-ray is taken, the patient should be told to take deep breaths to encourage generalized relaxation of his body. He should be reassured that feelings of warmth or a salty taste are often experienced by the patient when the dye is being injected and that this is transitory. The patient's face may even appear flushed at that time. If the patient manifests symptoms of respiratory distress, breaks out in a cold sweat, begins to feel clammy to the touch, and/or develops urticaria, an untoward reaction to the dye is occurring. In like manner, the patient complaining of a sensation of numbness or of palpitations should be observed carefully while the doctor is being notified. Many institutions require the injection of an antihistaminic prior to performance of the procedure; others specify that a syringe, needle, and medication accompany the patient to the x-ray department. Whatever the routine, the student should make certain that oxygen and an antihistamine drug can be readily mobilized for use in case of an emergency. Subsequent to the procedure, the student should force fluids—unless contraindicated because of associated disease—to help flush residual amounts of the dye from the urinary tract. The period of dehydration which is part of the preparation for the x-ray examination may also be countered by the forcing of fluids.

Cystoscopy refers to the procedure through which the bladder may be viewed directly and the ureters catheterized; this is accomplished with an instrument called a *cystoscope* (see Fig. 4), which is passed transurethrally. The cystoscope consists of four parts: the sheath, the obturator, the observation lens, and the working lens. The *sheath* or outermost cylinder is hollow and made of metal; it is the part which is passed through the urethra and into the bladder. The sheath comes in various sizes, much the same as catheters. The *obturator* is a solid, metal cylinder which is inserted into the sheath and passed transurethrally with it. The *observation lens* contains mirrors and lenses which allow the urologist to visualize the bladder, hence its name. After the sheath and obturator have been passed, the obturator is removed and the observation lens is inserted. If previous culture of urine from the bladder has revealed a significant bacterial count and the urologist

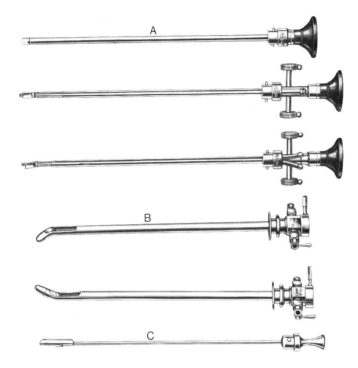

Fig. 4. The cystoscope. A. Telescopes. Three types of telescopes (or lenses) are shown: (from top downward) the examining, operating, and double catheterizing telescopes. B. Sheaths. A concave and convex sheath are shown. C. The obturator fits both sheaths. (Courtesy of American Cystoscope Makers, Inc., Pelham Manor, New York.)

wants to ascertain if bacteria are also present in urine of the upper urinary tract, catheterization of the ureters is necessary. The *working lens* of the cystoscope will make this possible, and it may be used instead of the observation lens. The working lens has channels through which ureteral catheters may be inserted and threaded upward through the ureteral orifices and into the ureters. With the ureteral catheters threaded into the kidney pelves, after urine specimens have been obtained, a retrograde *pyelogram* may be done if desired. When more clearly defined x-rays of the urinary collecting system (kidney pelves, calyces, ureters, and bladder) are desired to confirm the findings of an IVP or—in instances in which an IVP is contraindicated, retrograde pyelography may be used to provide the essential data needed. Radiopaque solution may be instilled via the ureteral catheters directly into the kidney pelves. This will outline the contour of the pelves and calyces. As the medium is carried downward in the urinary tract by the peristaltic waves of the ureters, an x-ray film is taken. In this manner the position and caliber of the lumen of both ureters as well as the contour of the badder may be evaluated. Retrograde films usually provide more definition and clarity than IVP films because the dye does not have to circulate in the blood or be excreted into the kidney pelves.

The student should remember that "*oscopy*" is *a visualization of*, while a *scope* provides the means by which such visualization may be accomplished. The prefix usually informs the reader about the cavity which is to be viewed. (Thus a cystoscope makes visualization of the bladder possible; a urethroscope, the urethra; a proctoscope, the rectum, etc.) Often endoscopy will be done. The endoscope is similar to the cystoscope but it is shorter and has no working lens. However, the endoscope will allow the urologist to make observations of the urethra and of prostatic enlargement about the bladder neck. An instrument which provides the means by which a resection may be accomplished is called a *resectoscope;* the resectoscope is the instrument used for the closed method of surgical treatment of benign prostatic hypertrophy. It is similar to the cystoscope (see Fig. 5), except that the working lens is equipped with channels for cutting and catheterizing loops to allow for resection and control of bleeders, respectively.

At the time that the consent forms are being signed, the nurse should ascertain how much the patient has been told about the procedure. If his knowledge is limited, the nurse may take the opportunity to prepare him for what will be done. A specific period of time will usually be designated when food

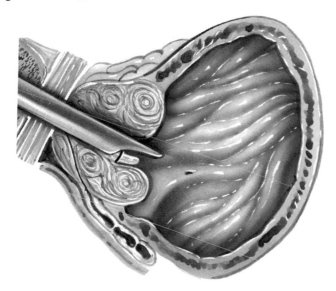

Fig. 5. The resectoscope. Note the cutting wire at the tip of the resectoscope. This accomplishes tissue resection within the bladder. (From Roen. Atlas of Urologic Surgery. 1967. Courtesy of Appleton-Century-Crofts.)

is to be withheld. Generally fluids may be forced for several hours prior to cystoscopy to assure excretion of urine by the kidneys during the procedure. In some hospitals, cystoscopy is performed in the x-ray department. In others, the procedure is done in the operating suite in a room specifically designated for that purpose. When anesthesia is to be used, IV fluids are given to assure urinary flow. The patient is usually medicated before the procedure (because a metal instrument is to be passed), and the patient is placed in lithotomy position. If present during the procedure, the student should make sure that the patient is adequately draped; and when the patient remains awake and seems apprehensive, he should be encouraged to take slow, deep breaths that will often effect relaxation. Words of empathy and reassurance often prove helpful in this situation.

After the cystoscope has been inserted, the bladder is

usually distended with sterile water or saline. A small electric bulb within the instrument provides the light which facilitates visualization of the bladder wall and ureteral orifices. Fluid within the bladder may be evacuated or instilled at the urologist's discretion. When ureteral catheters are used, urine may be collected from each kidney pelvis for analysis and bacteriologic study. The student should be careful to label the collecting tubes correctly: left kidney, right kidney.

The patient is usually kept on bedrest for a specified period of time following cystoscopy. He should be encouraged to force fluids and, generally, may be given pain medication as needed. The primary responsibility of the student during this interval is that of observation for signs of *anuria, hematuria, chills,* and/or *fever.* The doctor should be notified if the patient fails to void within an 8-hour period following the procedure. If the patient does void, the urine should be observed for blood since trauma secondary to instrumentation may have occurred. Complaints of a chill should alert the student to take the patient's temperature because chills often herald the presence of infection. The nurse's notes should include mention of the character of the first voided specimen and whether the patient has been febrile or afebrile following the procedure.

Significant blood chemistries included in the diagnostic work-up of patients with benign hypertrophy of the prostate gland are urea nitrogen (BUN) and nonprotein nitrogen (NPN) determinations. A patient may be *azotemic* (i.e., have elevated levels of nitrogenous waste in the blood) without manifesting symptoms. Such laboratory values provide an index to the degree of renal impairment (if any) that may be present. Further, since many patients present with undiagnosed associated disease, a fasting blood sugar (FBS) is routinely done. Diabetes mellitus may be discovered in patients within the age group usually affected by benign hypertrophy of the prostate.

An evaluation of the patient's general physical status would be incomplete without careful examination of the cardiovascular system. Nocturia and/or episodes of polyuria due to paroxysmal tachycardia must be ruled out. Then, after all pertinent testing has been completed, the determining factor for the type of surgical intervention that will be employed is the patient's overall physical condition and the status of his renal function. To complete the clinical picture, a phenolsulfonphthalein test (PSP) may be done. The PSP test measures renal tubular function. The student usually encourages the patient to drink two or more glasses of water (approximately 400 ml after which 1 ml of phenolsulfonphthalein is injected intravenously. (Intramuscular injection is sometimes given in lieu of IV administration.) When the dye has been given, urine specimens are collected at half-hourly intervals for 2 hours. Specimens of 100 ml or more each half hour will assure a satisfactory test. The percentage of phenolsulfonphthalein excreted during the 2-hour period delineates the functioning ability of the kidneys.

CARE OF THE PATIENT WITH CHRONIC URINARY RETENTION

Relief for the patient with acute retention is usually provided by immediate catheterization to effect emptying of the bladder and the alleviation of pain. In this situation, the rapid evacuation of the bladder is not likely to cause untoward reactions. An indwelling catheter attached to a straight or vented gravity drainage system (see Chapter 3) may be left in place thereafter and the preoperative evaluation of the patient begun. The management of chronic retention, however, poses a more complex problem. Since larger volumes of retained urine are usually involved (sometimes exceeding 1 to $1\frac{1}{2}$ liters), rapid evacuation of the bladder might cause gross hematuria second-

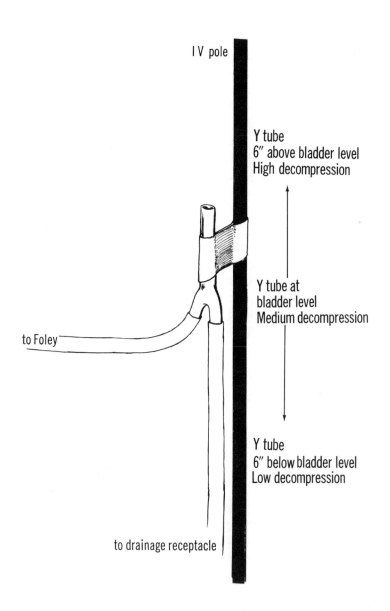

Fig. 6. The decompression drainage set-up.

ary to the sudden release of pressure on distended prostatic veins. Therefore, when the patient has a history of chronic urinary retention or when the bladder is greatly distended, a decompression drainage system is required (see Chapter 3). This will provide a gradual decompression of the bladder because outflowing urine is channeled contrary to the pull of gravity before it drains into the collecting receptacle. Hematuria may occur, but usually it will not be copious.

Insertion of an indwelling catheter may be difficult in the case of chronic retention, depending on the degree of prostatic enlargement and/or the amount of constriction of the prostatic urethra in the patient. If difficulty is encountered, a filiform may be inserted into a markedly narrowed outlet and a follower attached to accomplish drainage of the distended bladder (see Chapter 3). Since the follower is not a self-retaining catheter, the doctor will secure it in place with adhesive tape after it has been attached to the drainage apparatus. Initially, the follower may be attached to a medium or high decompression drainage system, depending on the degree of distention (see Fig. 6). If decremental decompression is desired, the Y-tube of the decompression drainage system may be lowered a specified number of inches at specified intervals until the bladder is completely decompressed. An order might read:

> Attach follower to high decompression drainage.
> Then lower Y-tube 6 in. q shift x 2. Attach follower to straight gravity drainage thereafter.

Thus, high, medium, and low decompression may be utilized in the evacuation of the markedly distended bladder. The filiform and follower (see Fig. 7) are seldom allowed to remain in place longer than 72 hours because the filiform may cause irritation and/or trauma to the bladder wall when it is no longer distended. By that time the follower has usually dilated the passageway sufficiently to allow the passage of a self-retain-

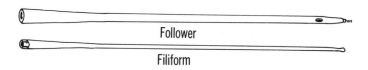

Fig. 7. The Philips dilator. When inserted, the filiform conforms to the contour of the bladder, curving somewhat so that its length is accommodated. The follower accomplishes the drainage of the bladder.

ing catheter and is replaced by it. After the retention has been resolved, the doctor may want periodic cleansing of the bladder or topical administration of antibacterial medication to treat a bladder infection. In such instances, an intermittent bladder irrigation set-up may be ordered.

The primary responsibility of the student in the care of the patient with acute or chronic retention is proper maintenance of the aforementioned inflow (irrigation) and outflow (drainage) systems. *They must be set up properly.* In order to do this, the student should understand the rationale for the utilization of the drainage of irrigating system and have knowledge of the principle underlying its functioning. Maintenance also involves observation of the drainage tubing and catheter care as previously discussed in Chapter 3. It should be stressed, however, that—although such work is preferably carried out by an orderly—daily care of the tissue immediately surrounding the catheter at the urethral orifice is a *nursing responsibility.* Inspection should be done with much the same attitude that is assumed when any treatment is to be done. The *catheter* may be gently manipulated to facilitate complete visualization. When an orderly is available, he should be instructed to inspect the area for dryness, cleanliness, and signs of swelling. The student should remember that *daily cleansing* reduces the possibility of infection, and this fact should be impressed on ancillary personnel. Crusts and exudate which tend to collect around the catheter at the urethral orifice should be removed and a thin film of Vaseline or cold cream may be placed on the tissue of that area to protect it from excoriation and to facilitate any subsequent removal of foreign matter.

CONSERVATIVE TREATMENT OF THE PATIENT

Conservative treatment of the patient with benign prostatic hypertrophy is concerned with relieving the acute symptoms of the patient. Many patients complaining of the symptoms of prostatism may be relieved by periodic medical treatment. This course of intervention, however, bears a direct relationship to the degree of vesical neck obstruction and to the age and general physical status of the patient. Not every case will be severe enough to warrant surgical intervention; not every patient will be able to withstand prostatic surgical procedures.

Prostatic massage and hot sitz baths are the treatments of choice for some patients. Prostatic massage causes small amounts of prostatic fluid to be released from the gland. Hot sitz baths are believed to accelerate prostatic circulation thereby increasing the rate of reabsorption of the released fluid. These treatment modalities, when used in conjunction, tend to reduce edema in the prostate. With an index finger inserted into the rectum, the lateral borders of the prostate may be massaged by the urologist. Initially, this treatment is usually done on a weekly basis. Thereafter, the intervals between treatments may be extended, depending on the duration of the patient's relief from symptoms. The 20-minute hot sitz bath is usually prescribed for alternate nights, the frequency being reduced as symptoms improve. As a result of this combination therapy, the patient usually urinates less frequently and notes a larger stream. He also has less difficulty in starting the stream, and often the amount of residual urine decreases.

For some patients bladder neck dilatation will effect relief of the symptoms of prostatism. Bougies, large catheters, or sounds may be used to dilate the prostatic urethra and the bladder neck. However, the risk of trauma and/or subsequent acute retention is great if the patient has a markedly weakened stream and a large urinary residual. Therefore, this course of treatment is usually undertaken in younger patients with a small degree of hypertrophy and little or no residual urine.

In addition to the modalities already mentioned, the nurse may advise the patient to limit fluid intake in the late evening as a means of reducing nocturnal frequency. He should be told not to drink large quantities of fluid at one time and should also be cautioned to empty his bladder before going out in cold weather. Symptoms seem to abate in warm weather.

SURGICAL INTERVENTION AS THE TREATMENT MODALITY OF CHOICE

Some of the indications for surgical intervention in the care of the patient with benign prostatic hypertrophy are a large residual urine, bladder and upper urinary tract changes, bladder changes alone, sequelae of increased intraabdominal pressure such as hernia (hemorrhoids may also develop as a result of the patient's straining to start his urinary stream), and uncontrollable hemorrhage. Infarction within the prostate will lead to hemorrhaging and removal of the hyperplastic tissue will leave a smooth lining in which bleeding can be more easily controlled. (When the periurethral tissue hypertrophies, normal tissue is pushed laterally toward the prostatic capsule. The pressure from the enlargement causes atrophy of the normal prostatic tissue and a "false capsule" or capsule within the capsule is formed. *The atrophied normal tissue plus the prostatic capsule form a lateral boundary which encloses the hyperplastic tissue.* It is understandable, then, how hyperplastic tissue may be enucleated or peeled from its bed inside the atrophied tissue wall formed by its growth.)

As previously stated, the preoperative nursing care of these patients includes the setting up of the urinary drainage apparatus; catheter care and care of the urinary drainage tubing; the forcing of fluids; insuring adequate rest and ambulation of the patient; and the preparation and after-care of the patient during the various stages of the diagnostic work-up. There are four standard approaches that may be used for the removal of the hypertrophied portion of the gland: the transurethral approach, the suprapubic approach, the retropubic approach, and the perineal approach. The preoperative work-up helps the doctors choose the one best suited to the needs of the patient. The age and condition of the patient, the size and location of the gland, and the presence of associated disease are the factors which usually determine the operative approach that the urologist will choose. A new technique which utilizes the transurethral approach—*cryosurgery*—is currently being evaluated.

Bilateral Vasectomy

In patients requiring surgical intervention for relief of the symptoms of prostatism, *bilateral vasectomy* is routinely done as a prophylactic measure against the possibility of infectious organisms (from the prostatic cavity and urethra) refluxing down the vas deferens and causing epididymitis following prostatectomy. Simple vas ligation preceding all prostatectomy operations has proved to be inadequate for the prevention of this inflammatory process. Often during the second postoperative week patients developed high fever secondary to acute infection of the epididymis. Investigation of the method yielded valuable information because animal experimentation demonstrated that, following ligation, patency of the vas was often reestablished. Since restricted activity is an essential part of the treatment of epididymitis the patient is subjected to the possibility of developing phlebitis, an embolism, a myocardial infarction (especially the aged, debilitated patient), and/or other complications. Hospitalization is also extended. Thus partial vasectomy has currently become the procedure of choice for the prevention of postprostatectomy epididymitis.

A small incision is made on either side of the upper scrotal region and approximately 2 cm of the spermatic passageway is excised. This is followed by ligation of the severed ends and suturing of the scrotal incisions. Healing usually proceeds uneventfully. The patient will be sterile following the procedure, but this is seldom of consequence to patients in the age group affected by benign hypertrophy of the prostate. However, when there is strong feeling against the procedure, the patient should be told that he faces the discomfort and prolonged hospitalization associated with epididymitis if it develops, and that the amount of semen ejaculated is greatly diminished after prostatectomy because ejacuation refluxes into the bladder.

Transurethral Prostatectomy

Transurethral resection of the prostate gland is best employed when a small to moderate degree of hypertrophy exists. Patients prefer it to other methods utilized for the removal of the hypertrophied part of the gland. No incision is necessary. There is also less postoperative discomfort, immobilization, and disability. In preparation for the procedure, the patient is placed in lithotomy position and his body is grounded against electrical shock through some specified manner which may vary from institution to institution. After a resectoscope has been introduced transurethrally, small pieces of hyperplastic tissue may be removed with an electric-wire cutting device (see Fig. 8).

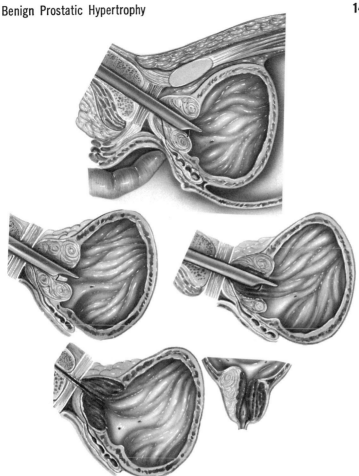

Fig. 8. Transurethral prostatic resection. The hypertrophied tissue is removed segment by segment. (From Roen. Atlas of Urologic Surgery. 1967. Courtesy of Appleton-Century-Crofts.)

In addition, the resectoscope accommodates a cauterizing attachment which accomplishes the control of bleeding. Thus, under direct vision afforded by the ocular device of the resectoscope, obstructive tissue may be completely removed. A continuous flow of irrigation solution throughout the operation insures clear visualization. An isotonic electrolyte solution such as sterile saline is *not* used during the operative irrigation because the electrolyte would diffuse current from the wire loop, thereby preventing it from cutting.

With the transurethral approach to prostatic surgery, there is always the possibility of trauma to the urethra from the resectoscope. Thus urethral stricture is more likely to occur following transurethral resection than any of the other three procedures. In addition, during the operation large prostatic veins are opened and the possibility of irrigating solutions' entering these veins and causing hemolysis* is always present—especially as sterile water is so frequently used as the irrigating solution during operation. (The student should be aware that the *hemoglobinemia* resulting from hemolysis can lead to renal failure, so that observations should be made for signs of cyanosis, jaundice, disorientation, and/or stupor in the early postoperative period. Skin color, the presence of specific areas of cyanosis—periorbital or in the nail beds—and the state of the patient's mental acuity should always be included in the nurse's notes made postoperatively.) Renal insufficiency and urethral stricture are possible untoward reactions to transurethral prostatectomy. It may be appreciated, therefore, why the patient's preference for this approach is seldom the determining factor when a urologist is choosing the surgical procedure for prostatic conditions. The transurethral procedure is usually the operation of choice when the patient is aged, infirmed, or a poor operative risk. The student may notice that some urologists will attempt to induce diuresis in these patients by ordering injections of mannitol before and during the operation. This is a precaution against the occurrence of increased

---

* It should be remembered that *hemolysis* is the separation of the hemoglobin from the red blood corpuscles, which results from the entrance into the circulation of either distilled water or water containing blood already hemolyzed in the bladder. The subsequent hemoglobinemia may result in renal failure—especially in patients with a history of renal impairment.

amounts of fluid circulating in the blood secondary to fluid entering the circulation via the venous sinus during surgical intervention.

After the operation a three-way Foley catheter is often inserted into the bladder. One channel of the catheter allows for inflation of the self-retaining balloon. A constant bladder irrigation set-up is usually connected to the "inflow" channel of the catheter, with urinary drainage tubing being connected to the "outflow" channel. Sterile water is not used as the postoperative bladder irrigating solution because of the danger of hemolysis when significant amounts of water enter the circulation. Saline is also not used during this immediate postoperative period because entrance of significant amounts of an isotonic irrigating solution into the venous sinus of the prostate could initiate cardiac failure. In many hospitals, 2½ percent glucose in water is the solution of choice during the postoperative irrigation period. However, even when this precaution is taken, the student should still be aware of some of the signs and symptoms of cardiorenal insufficiency: hypertension, mental confusion, nausea and vomiting, edema, and weight gain. *Restriction of fluid intake is indicated in this instance.*

A gravity drainage system is usually ordered for the "outflow channel; however, decompression drainage may be requested. The student should realize that decompression drainage in this instance would be ordered to provide hemostasis by insuring the maintenance of constant pressure at the bladder neck (from retained urine). The bladder is prevented from emptying completely (as is the case with the gravity drainage system), and the intravesical urinary level must reach a certain height before there will be enough internal pressure to force urine out of the bladder and up the short arm of the inverted Y-tube against the pull of gravity. Further, a constant fluid level in the bladder tends to decrease the severity of bladder spasms.

Observation for evidence of hemorrhage is a primary

nursing responsibility during the early postoperative period. The urinary drainage is usually quite bloody, but the vital signs will be a good index to the patient's status. The constant bladder irrigation tends to control bleeding, which gradually subsides as healing takes place. A few patients may experience mild febrile reactions secondary to the procedure, but *no rectal temperatures should be taken.* Because of the proximity of the rectum to the operative site, rectal treatments (eg., taking temperatures and/or giving enemas) are discouraged as bleeding could easily occur. If bladder spasms are experienced, they usually represent the bladder's attempt to expel retained clots. These clots may be expressed under pressure with an asepto syringe (as described in the study at the end of this chapter) if the tubing becomes clogged and attempts to clear the lumen by "milking" of the tubing prove unsuccessful.

The prevention of postoperative atelectasis is an equally important nursing responsibility. Even with the extraabdominal operative approach and the minimal postoperative pain which is characteristic of the transurethral procedure, many of the patients have difficulty in coughing to forcibly remove bronchial secretions. The student will also discover that many elderly patients tend to have degenerative pulmonary changes; therefore, spinal anesthesia is frequently used because ordinarily this route of administration will not adversely affect respiratory function. In addition to early ambulation, the patient should be encouraged to take deep breaths as an aid in preventing atelectasis.

The indwelling catheter may remain in place from three to seven days postoperatively. Subsequent to the removal of the catheter, a record of the time and amount of each voiding should be kept. The patient will usually be discharged shortly thereafter if no further bleeding is noted and if urinary function progresses uneventfully. Transitory incontinence after the removal of the catheter may occur because of an associated bladder infection or incomplete wound healing. The patient will complain of experiencing a sudden desire to void, and he becomes incontinent because of the urgency. This "urgency incontinence" tends to resolve itself as healing progresses and infection subsides. Prior to discharge the patient should be told that he may experience occasional episodes of scant bleeding during urination. He should be informed that these experiences may occur two to four weeks after operation and that they are caused by the sloughing of coagulated prostatic tissue. Then he should be reassured that he need become concerned only if active bleeding occurs. To complete his preparation for discharge, he should be advised to force fluids (12 to 14 glasses daily) for at least a month and to refrain from doing excessive work for at least three weeks following discharge.

Occasionally after the catheter has been removed a patient will have difficulty voiding and will retain moderate amounts of urine in the bladder. The student will become aware of this early if accurate accounts of intake and the time and amount of output are kept. In such cases, factors other than inadequate operative technique (such as lack of bladder tone secondary to chronic retention, or neurologic changes secondary to the aging process) may be the cause. For such patients, an indwelling catheter may be reinserted before they are discharged. Since the catheter will remain in situ until the bladder tone returns, instructing the patient regarding catheter care and personal hygiene is essential during the predischarge period. Enough time should be allotted for supervision of self-care so that the patient's confidence may be built up. Modifications of technique to approximate home conditions should be discussed.

Postoperative stricture and/or bladder neck contracture are usually treated by dilatation with a filiform and a succession of followers (graduated in size) until the outlet is adequately dilated. Sounds may also be used for dilatation and periodic sounding may be necessary thereafter to maintain an adequate outlet.

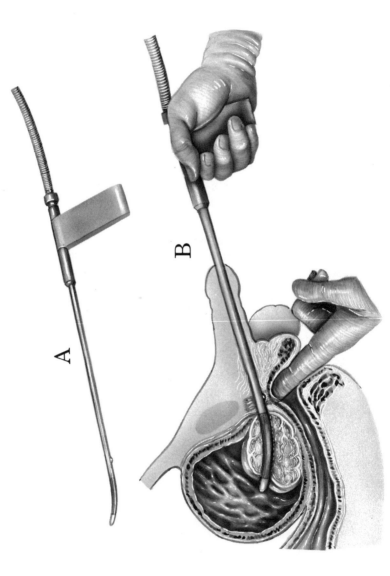

Fig. 9AB. Cryosurgery of the prostate. A. The probe has a 26 Fr diameter and is shaped like a sound. B. The projecting metal protuberance anterior to the examining finger is positioned so that the cooling segment of the probe is in the pro-

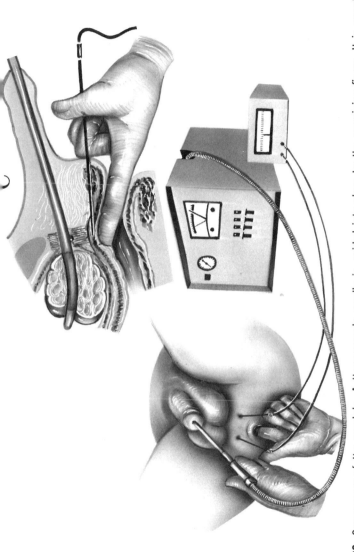

FIG. 9C. Cryosurgery of the prostate. A thermocouple needle is guided into place by the examining finger. It is sometimes placed in the prostatic capsule also. Activation of the cooling unit thereafter accomplishes the freezing of the prostate. (From Roen. Atlas of Urologic Surgery. 1967. Courtesy of Appleton-Century-Crofts.)

Cryosurgery of the Prostate

A new method of treatment for benign hypertrophy and/or carcinoma of the prostate gland is currently under investigation: *cryosurgery of the prostate.* The principle underlying the procedure is that ultrafreezing of prostatic tissue leads to intracellular changes which will destroy early carcinoma; the procedure is also indicated for the relief of bladder neck obstruction which is secondary to the growth of a prostatic neoplasm. When carcinoma of the prostate is suspected, a tissue biopsy must precede cryosurgery.

The transurethral approach is utilized for the insertion of a prostatic probe—an instrument shaped like a urethral sound (see Fig. 9a). The instrument is insulated so that only the distal section that comes in contact with the gland attains temperatures below the freezing level. (Probe temperatures lower than $-160°C$ can be attained, but the temperature within the periprostatic tissue is seldom reduced below the $-10°C$ level.) Liquid nitrogen accomplishes the freezing process and the instrument contains channels for its inflow and outflow. The probe is also equipped with a heating channel which causes thawing of the freezing section so that the instrument may be removed after maximum freezing of the tissue has been effected. The depth of freezing reached in the prostatic capsule and in the periprostatic tissue is monitored by thermocouple needles which are connected to a temperature gauge (see Figs. 9b and c). The needles are inserted transperineally and positioned under the guidance of an examining finger that is placed in the rectum. The depth of freezing attained in the probe is monitored by the cryosurgical cooling unit.

After the probe has been inserted and positioned correctly, the thermocouple needles are inserted into the prostatic capsule. Activation of the cryosurgical unit initiates and maintains the flow of nitrogen which accomplishes the freezing of the gland. The bladder wall is kept away from the area being frozen by air, which is introduced prior to undertaking the procedure. The length of time required for the freezing of the tissue varies according to the size of the gland, but usually freezing is accomplished in less than 10 minutes. Thereafter, the nitrogen flow is discontinued and the heating mechanism is activated just long enough to effect thawing so that the probe can be removed. Subsequent to the removal of the probe, a catheter is inserted into the bladder. It usually remains in place for about a week during that period of prostatic uretha rigidity that occurs secondary to the freezing process. Intracellular dehydration and cellular membrane rupture leads to the destruction of prostatic tissue. Although cryosurgery is a simple method which avoids the hazards of bleeding, a major disadvantage is that sloughing of the necrotic tissue may interfere with voiding after the catheter has been removed. In such instances, bladder irrigations are necessary to eliminate the sloughing tissue. This involves the recatheterization of the patient as well as prolonged hospitalization. Further, asymmetrical enlargement may pose a problem because sections of larger lobes may escape freezing and thereby retain their ability to hypertrophy. Thus, obstruction subsequent to cryosurgery may occur.

It would seem that cryosurgery is particularly suitable for the poorer risk patients because it is safe and can be done in a short period of time. However, clinical data regarding this new method are limited and further evaluation is currently being made.

Suprapubic prostatectomy

Suprapubic prostatectomy permits blunt enucleation of the prostate gland and inspection of the bladder for pathologic processes such as calculi and tumors. Through a small incision in the abdominal area above the pubic bone, the rectus muscles are separated and the anterior surface of the bladder is incised near the bladder neck. After inspection, the surgeon inserts an index finger into the bladder neck and urethra. The surgeon may or may not insert a finger of his other hand into the rectum to push the gland anteriorly. The mucous membrane surrounding the anterior part of the hypertrophied tissue is split. The line of cleavage between the hypertrophied lobe and the false capsule is located and the hyperplastic tissue is removed by blunt finger dissection (see Fig. 10). When other obstructing lobes have been similarly removed and bleeding vessels at the bladder neck ligated, packing (hemostatic material) may be placed into the prostatic fossa. Packing is not always used however. A Foley catheter may also be inserted at this time and—after it is inflated—the balloon may be pulled down into the prostatic cavity to act as a tamponade. Traction on the balloon is obtained by taping the catheter to the thigh for a few hours. Standard wound closure completes the procedure and a catheter is left to drain the bladder suprapubically (a suprapubic or *cystostomy* tube). The cystostomy tube is usually not a self-retaining catheter and must be held in place by an incisional suture.

Although suprapubic prostatectomy is usually carried out as a one-stage procedure, two stages are often required in patients who show an elevated blood urea nitrogen, a severe bladder infection, or a general debilitating disease accompanying the prostatic obstruction. The two-stage method consists of cystostomy drainage of the bladder for 10 to 14 days until the patient's general condition improves and subsequent prostatic enucleation by either the suprapubic or transurethral approach can be done. Local anesthesia is usually employed for the insertion of the suprapubic tube. The two-stage method is especially applicable for the uremic patient or when a

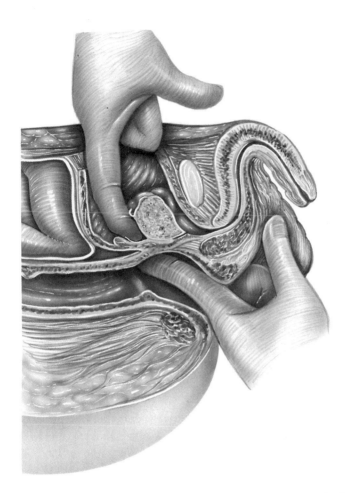

Fig. 10. Suprapubic enucleation of the prostate. Note how the hypertrophied tissue is bluntly cored out by the surgeon's finger. (From Roen. Atlas of Urologic Surgery. 1967. Courtesy of Appleton-Century-Crofts.)

urethral catheter cannot be inserted. If prolonged cystostomy drainage is necessary and the suprapubic route is to be utilized for the second stage, the fistulous suprapubic tract must be excised before closure. Usually less bleeding will be noted following the second procedure of the two-stage prostatectomy because the initial period of urinary drainage tends to diminish vascular congestion in the gland.

Suprapubic prostatectomy is technically simple to perform and requires neither special instruments nor exaggerated positioning of the patient. It can be employed for the removal of a large gland, regardless of its position within the pelvis. Concurrent treatment of associated lesions within the bladder can be done. However, most urologists agree that it should not be employed for the removal of small fibrotic glands. It should also be stated that the disadvantage of surgical interruption of the bladder musculature is present and this technique is associated with great blood loss. Further urinary leakage around the cystostomy tube poses the possibility of skin irritation and excoriation, and the extended period of convalescence is fraught with intervals of great discomfort. Bladder spasms characteristically follow suprapubic enucleation of the prostate. In medicating the patient with an analgesic (or anti-spasmodic when severe episodes have warranted such an order) the student should instruct the patient to refrain from "bearing down" to urinate by taking *slow, deep breaths*. This will aid in relaxation and will tend to decrease the intensity of the spasm. Ingestion of warm liquids also tends to diminish the severity of the spasms. When the patient complains of bladder spasms, observation of the drainage tubing should be made to insure that spasms are not a result of faulty drainage flow. Sluggish drainage and complaints of spasms in the early postoperative period are usually due to clot retention in the bladder. The clots should be expressed under pressure exerted by an asepto syringe during a bladder irrigation. Although the spasms cause varying degrees of discomfort, depending on the individual, they seldom last longer than 72 hours after operation.

After the patient has been returned to the unit, the doctor's orders *and* the operative note should be reviewed so that a *relevant postoperative nursing plan* may be devised. The cystostomy tube is usually connected to a gravity drainage system and the student may expect grossly bloody drainage. The vital signs should be used as an index to assist in the differentiation between characteristic postoperative bleeding following suprapubic prostatectomy and hemorrhage. The dressing should be checked thereafter and reinforced if excessive drainage is noted; *it should not be changed initially by the nursing staff* because accidental dislodgement of the packing may cause hemorrhage. The student will often note sanguinous drainage leaking from the urethra, especially if a Foley catheter has not been inserted during the operation. The groin, scrotum, and perineal region should be cleansed of dried blood (which will probably be present), and clean compresses may be placed so as to absorb subsequent urethral drainage. This cleansing is a *nursing* responsibility and gloves may be donned when an orderly is not available and the student must perform the treatment. In most instances the patient will be unable to perform this self-care because of drowsiness from medication and/or inability to bend forward to reach the area because of the placement of the cystostomy tube. The sutures that will be noted in the upper, anterior scrotal area on either side will indicate that bilateral vasectomy has been performed.

The initial dressing change and removal of the packing from the prostatic fossa are usually done early on the first postoperative day. The patient is encouraged to ambulate progressively thereafter. It should be appreciated that discomfort from the cystostomy tube will cause the patient to hesitate when movement is encouraged, and empathy from the nurse is in order. However, it should be remembered that patients in this age group are particularly susceptible to embolism and hypostatic pneumonia—thus the student must assume a gentle but firm approach in encouraging turning, coughing, deep breathing, and early ambulation. A word of caution seems appropriate at this juncture. An order for the patient to be assisted out of bed and into a chair means just that. The patient should not be encouraged to walk about at that time. Such premature movement may increase the amount of bleeding from the prostatic cavity.

Dressings should be changed as often as necessary and the character and amount of drainage on the dressing should be recorded in the nurse's notes. Since the drainage present will represent bloody urinary drainage leaking out around the cystostomy tube, the term *urosanguinous drainage* will be applicable. The skin area around the tube must be cleansed *at each dressing change* and two things must be remembered. First of all, the student should take care to lift the cystostomy tube *gently* when attempting to clean the area beneath it. Any movement of the tube may initiate a spasm or otherwise cause discomfort to the patient. Secondly, cleansing strokes should be directed from the area immediately surrounding the cystostomy, down the suture line, and then outward onto the intact skin area. This technique will prevent bacteria and other contaminants from being swept from the skin area into the healing wound edges or into the raw area surrounding the tube, which would predispose the patient to infection. *Cleansing strokes should never be directed from the skin area toward the incisional area.*

The forcing of fluids during the postoperative period is essential, but iced fluids should be restricted: they tend to increase the incidence of bladder spasm. Rectal thermometers and rectal tubes should not be inserted because of the possibility of traumatizing the adjacent operative area and causing increased bleeding. Finally, patients should be advised not to strain to force a bowel movement: the pressure created will also cause bleeding to recur once it has subsided.

The cystostomy tube usually remains in place until the urine clears—from 3 to 5 days. A Foley catheter is inserted thereafter and remains in place to drain the bladder until the suprapubic wound has healed (if one has not been inserted at the time of operation). After the cystostomy tube has been removed, large amounts of *urinary drainage* should be anticipated and frequent dressing changes should be done. The amount of suprapubic drainage will diminish as healing progresses, and the patient will usually be ready for discharge within 21 postoperative days. At the time of discharge, if a small suprapubic sinus persists because of incomplete healing, the patient or his family may be advised to place a small compress over the area (secured with scotch tape to prevent excoriation of the skin as a result of daily changes). Patients are usually permitted to take tub baths as the warm water stimulates the circulation and this assists the healing process.

Retropubic prostatectomy

Retropubic prostatectomy is especially suitable for large glands which are situated high in the pelvis. This surgical method is accomplished through a low abdominal incision (see Fig. 11a). The gland is approached between the pubic arch and the bladder. With the anterior surface of the gland exposed, the *prostatic capsule* is incised and the hypertrophied part of the gland is enucleated. This method allows for the ligation or fulguration of bleeders under direct vision. A Foley catheter is inserted transurethrally after the hyperplastic tissue has been removed and, when the self-retaining balloon has been inflated, the catheter is pulled downward into the prostatic fossa at the bladder neck to aid in hemostatis. Subsequently, the anterior prostatic capsule is sutured and the wound closed.

Although the incidence of osteitis pubis (inflammation of the pubic bone) following this type of operation has diminished, the possibility of its occurrence still exists. The patient

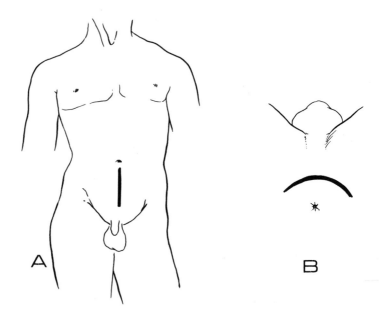

Fig. 11. A. Incisional site for the retropubic prostatectomy. B. Incisional site for the perineal prostatectomy. A low abdominal incision affords a retropubic approach to the prostate gland, whereas an incision behind the scrotum and in front of the anus accomplishes a perineal approach.

afflicted with this condition usually complains of severe pain which radiates down the inner aspect of one or both legs. Such complaints usually begin from 4 to 6 weeks after operation and the symptoms will usually be heralded by a fever. Extreme tenderness will be experienced when the symphysis pubis is palpated. As the inflammatory process continues, the patient will experience increasing difficulty in walking. Sitting also becomes painful if there is ischial involvement. The condition usually becomes resolved in time, but it can cause the patient great discomfort and in some instances has resulted in several months of disability. Remedial treatment usually involves administrations of cortisone and antibiotics, and the use of diathermy. The patient must also be afforded adequate rest and his activity should be limited. As a means of protecting the patient against the pain and discomfort of osteitis pubis, therefore, the surgeon always gives the space of Retzius (the space between the pubic bone and the bladder) a thorough cleansing prior to closure in order to effect the removal of clots and other debris. Since proper drainage is equally important, a drain is usually placed in the space.

Since the bladder is not incised in this surgical approach, patients experience less dysuria during their postoperative course; and, because the prostatic capsule heals more quickly than the bladder wall, there is a shorter period of convalescence following use of this technique. However, associated bladder disease cannot be treated when this approach is used. During the postoperative period, the student *should not expect to observe urinary drainage* on the dressing; small amounts of serosanguinous drainage may be noted. However, observation for signs and symptoms of hemorrhage is an important nursing responsibility. If bladder spasms are experienced by the patient, they will usually be mild, and he should be advised to take deep breaths when such spasms occur in order to avoid the urge to bear down and void. *After the drainage tubing is checked for patency* when such complaints arise, the patient should be reassured that the bladder is draining well and that the catheter is initiating the sensations he feels.

The drains are usually removed on the fourth postoperative day, but the catheter will usually remain in place for about a week. If minor episodes of postoperative bleeding occur, the catheter remains until the urine is clear. Urinary control following the removal of the catheter is seldom a problem.

Perineal prostatectomy

Perineal prostatectomy is the only method of prostatic enucleation which offers a direct anatomic approach to the prostate gland. A perineal prostatectomy is accomplished through a curved incision in the perineum (see Fig. 11b), which is located behind the scrotum and in front of the anus. The inferior surface of the prostatic capsule is incised and the hyperplastic tissue removed. Then, after the bleeders have been ligated, the capsule is closed and the perineal wound is sutured. A drain left in the perineum provides for necessary drainage of the area and the insertion of a Foley catheter completes the procedure. Since the patient must be placed in an exaggerated lithotomy position, perineal prostatectomy is unsuitable for patients with cardiac or respiratory impairment; however, the lowest incidence of postoperative hemorrhage and discomfort is associated with this procedure.

During the time that closed methods of biopsy were being investigated and evaluated, perineal prostatectomy was advantageous when open biopsy was indicated as a diagnostic aid for the determination of carcinomatous tissue. Currently, however, with the development of refined instruments and techniques for needle biopsy of the prostate, open surgical biopsy offers few advantages. The perineal approach is utilized more for radical surgery of the gland than for enucleation of benign hyperplastic tissue. The advantage of hemostasis under direct vision—resulting in the lower incidence of postoperative shock from hemorrhage—does not outweigh the disadvantages of this method. The perineal incision is usually deepened along the rectal wall to allow for exposure of the prostatic apex; thus danger of injury to the rectum is present. The possibility of direct injury to the urinary sphincter mechanism or of injury to the pudendal nerves is also present. Urinary incontinence secondary to such injury is a more likely complication of the perineal approach than of any of the other methods of enucleation. Further, impotence may also follow perineal prostatectomy.

The indwelling catheter and the perineal drain are usually removed within a week after operation. Bulky dressings may be indicated if a moderate amount of drainage is present. It should be remembered that the perineal route permits gravity drainage of the wound. A firm chair should be provided for the patient's comfort when he is ambulatory, but a rubber ring should be provided only with the doctor's permission.

Whatever the surgical approach to prostatic enucleation for benign hypertrophy, specific structural changes occur following prostatectomy. With improved urinary outflow, the complications of bladder neck obstruction (e.g., hydronephrosis and hydroureter) will begin to regress. Involution of the enlarged bladder musculature also occurs, and follow-up endoscopic examination in a year's time will often reveal the disappearance of trabeculations and the return of the characteristic smooth mucosa of the bladder wall. In some cases, as soon as six weeks after operation the normal caliber of the prostatic segment of the urethra returns. This is a result of the dual effects of the involution of the "true" capsule of the prostate (involution of the walls of the fossa created from prostatic enucleation) and the process of epithelization from the mucosa of the bladder neck and membranous urethra. The patient should be reminded to abstain from sexual intercourse for three months because of the possibility of hemorrhage secondary to congestion of the "true" capsule.

Following prostatectomy, the urine may continue to be infected for several weeks. During this interval, the patient may experience frequency, some degree of burning on urination, and episodes of incontinence resulting from the urgency associated with the sudden desire to urinate. The patient should be told to urinate at regular intervals during the day (e.g., every 3 hours or so) and not to wait until he has the urge to void. The drinking of 12 to 14 glasses of fluid daily will insure the presence of urine in the bladder. Regular evacuation will tend to exercise the external sphincter as well as prohibit the sudden, unexpected urge to void which may lead to urgency incontinence while the activity of the external sphincter is still sluggish. The patient should also be advised to restrict the intake of spicy foods and alcoholic beverages because of their irritating effect. Usually, the infection gradually subsides after the cause of the obstruction to the free outflow of urine has been removed. The external sphincter regains full control over continency. Symptoms of dysuria abate and the normal voiding patterns may be resumed. In cases of persistent infection, medical intervention is indicated and vigorous chemotherapeutic and/or antibiotic treatment may be required.

From two to three months postoperatively, follow-up examination will usually include catheterization for residual urine determination and urethral calibration to check for stricture or bladder neck contracture. If obstruction develops secondary to these conditions, appropriate treatment is instituted. It should be noted that, since none of the techniques discussed involves the removal of the prostatic capsule, hypertrophy subsequent to enucleation of hyperplastic tissue can develop.

A NURSING-CARE STUDY

Mr. P. is a 67-year-old man who consulted his doctor after experiencing progressive difficulty in starting his urinary stream when voiding. Some dribbling and dysuria were noted, and the force of the stream had diminished. Frequency of urination was also noted—the patient experienced nocturia an average of three to five times per night. These symptoms had progressed gradually over a six-month period prior to Mr. P.'s consultation with his doctor. The patient reported no history of hematuria, fever, chills, or calculi in the urinary tract. The rectal examination that was performed revealed an enlarged prostate gland which was firm, smooth, and regular. A tentative diagnosis of benign prostatic hypertrophy was made and Mr. P. subsequently entered the hospital for operation.

When the patient was admitted to the unit, a

student noted that he was in no apparent distress. After he was oriented to the unit, a urine specimen was collected and sent to the laboratory and the doctor was notified. The following orders were written after the history was taken and the admission physical completed:

CBC
Urine to lab
OOB ad lib
Diet as tolerated
Chest x-ray
EKG
For IVP: Permission
             Neoloid 90 ml @ 7 P.M.
             NPO after midnight
Serum acid phosphatase & serum alkaline phosphatase
     determinations
BUN and FBS in A.M.

A nurse witnessed the patient's signing of the permission form for the IVP after ascertaining that the doctor had discussed the treatment with him. It was further explained that a cathartic would be given so that the bowel would be empty and clear x-ray pictures obtained. The medication was given for the bowel preparation as ordered, and an NPO-after-midnight sign was taped *conspicuously* to the head of the bed. The patient understood that—in addition to the emptying of the bowel to eliminate cloudy x-ray films of the urinary collecting system— fluid restriction was also necessary to insure optimum visualization. The dye to be injected intravenously would circulate in a more concentrated form if he was slightly dehydrated.

The blood work was done the following morning as ordered, and the patient was taken for x-rays thereafter. (Serum phosphatases are ordered as routine screening tests—to rule out carcinoma—in every case of prostatic work-up.) Upon his return to the unit, the student conscientiously *forced fluids* to make up for the interval of restricted fluid intake and Mr.

P. tolerated this well. Frequency of voiding was noted and recorded, and the patient continued to complain of difficulty in starting and maintaining the urinary stream. The following day, after the x-ray reports were received on the unit and placed in the chart, the student assigned to his care noted that the chest film was normal; it was also noted that, although the IVP was grossly normal, an elevation within the bladder caused by an enlarged prostate was revealed and there was some urinary retention. Thus the tentative diagnosis of benign prostatic hypertrophy was substantiated and the following pre-operative orders were written:

X-match for 1,000 ml blood for OR in A.M.
Shave and prep for suprapubic prostatectomy
Permission to include bilateral vasectomy
NPO after midnight
Chloral hydrate 0/5 g h.s.
Na amytal 100 mg @ 11 A.M.
Atropine 0/3 mg (IM) on call

Before obtaining the patient's signature on the operative permit or having the patient shaved and the area scrubbed with surgical soap in preparation for suprapubic prostatectomy, the student discussed the forthcoming procedure with the patient to find out what he had been told by his doctor. Mr. P. understood that his prostate gland was to be removed through a suprapubic incision and that some "tubes were going to be tied." He knew this would make him sterile, but said that was of no consequence at his age. He did admit, however, that he couldn't quite visualize where these structures were or how they "blocked off the urine passageway." To clarify matters, therefore, the student drew a crude anatomic diagram of the prostate gland surrounding the bladder neck and of the adjacent vas deferens extending downward to the testicle. A simple explanation and illustration could then be given of how enlargement of the prostate gland had caused a narrowing of the urinary outlet. It was further shown that sterility occurred when the vas deferens was ligated because the passageway of the sperm would be blocked off. The patient seemed fascinated by the dynamics of the process and asked if he could keep the diagram.

The student then told the patient that he would have to cough and deep-breathe in the immediate postoperative period so that his lungs would not become congested and his hospital stay lengthened. Mr. P. was instructed to support the lower abdominal region with his hands, and he practiced taking deep breaths and coughing. The student also told the patient about the discomfort and "urge to void" that he would experience following surgery. It was explained that during surgery packing is placed in the space left after the prostate has been removed. The presence of packing and the cystostomy tube often cause patients to feel a continuous urge to void. (This can be extremely distressing in the immediate postoperative period if the patient has not been told about it during the preoperative period.) The team leader obtained his signature on the operative permit and the shave and prep was completed after the student reported that the patient had been told about the operation. Before the student left the clinical area, an NPO-after-midnight sign was again taped conspicuously on the patient's bed, and the next morning the patient was taken to the operating room.

The same student who had done the preoperative teaching was assigned to his postoperative care. When Mr. P. was returned to the unit at 4 P.M., he was glad to see the familiar face. After checking the IV to make sure it was running well, the nurse took the patient's vital signs (which were stable). His dressing was dry and intact, but some sanguinous drainage per urethra was noted. Clean abdominal pads were placed so as to absorb the drainage and the student would thus be able to report an estimate of the blood loss to the doctor: "two abdominal pads saturated with *sanguinous* drainage from the urethra were replaced × 2 during a 6-hour interval." Mr. P.'s only complaint was of the urge to void.

After the initial observations were made, the student reviewed the doctor's orders *and the operative note*. The following postoperative orders had been written:

Demerol 75 mg q 4 h (IM) for pain; give 75 mg @ 7 A.M. tomorrow—drains to be removed @ 7:30 A.M.

Change dressing PRN and cleanse area with surgical soap and alcohol and boric acid solution *after* drains are removed in A.M.

Place cystostomy tube to straight gravity drainage

Irrigate cystostomy tube only if absolutely necessary; tube may be irrigated PRN after drains are removed

Bedrest

Vital signs q 15 min × 4, q 30 min × 2, q1 h × 3, then q 2 h

NPO until 9 P.M., then allow hot tea/warm water/warm lemonade if no nausea

Record intake and output

Combiotic 2 ml (IM) BID

Hct 6 P.M. and 12 midnight

The operative note revealed that a suprapubic prostatectomy and bilateral vasectomy had been performed. There were three Penrose drains in the prostatic bed, and a right-angle, whistle-tip, 40 Fr catheter had been inserted into the bladder for drainage via the suprapubic incision—*the cystostomy tube*. Knowledge of the facts obtained from the operative note *and* the specifics of the immediate postoperative surgical-care plan (obtained from the doctor's order sheet) enabled the student *to develop a preliminary nursing-care plan* as well as to carry out the doctor's orders comprehensively.

The student returned to the patient's bedside and attached the cystostomy tube to a straight gravity set-up; the drainage was *urosanguinous*. (It should be remembered that *serosanguinous* would be inappropriate terminolgy for a description of bloody drainage derived from the bladder). Mr. P. was encouraged to cough and deep-breathe thereafter, and assisted in turning on his side; a pillow was placed along the length of his back for support and to maintain the position. The student checked to make sure that the patient was not lying on the drainage tubing and that the tubing ran straight into the collecting receptacle—without looping on itself after leaving the edge of the bed or hanging below the level of the collecting receptacle before entering it. A mouth-care tray consisting of a cup of glycerine and lemon juice, a cup of mouth wash, and a few tongue depressors covered with gauze compresses was then brought to the bedside so that dryness and/or complaints of "sour taste" could be relieved until that time when Mr. P. would be allowed fluids. His vital signs remained stable so he was given the medication ordered for the relief of his pain. Thereafter, he was encouraged to turn, cough, and deep-breathe every hour. At 9 P.M. he drank some warm tea since he had no complaints of nausea; he tolerated it well.

Although bleeding was anticipated, the student was concerned about the grossly bloody drainage. The clinical instructor was consulted, therefore, and it was agreed that the patient's pulse and blood pressure should be carefully observed so that anticipated bleeding following suprapubic enucleation of the prostate could be differentiated from postoperative hemorrhaging. The vital signs did not fluctuate, however. The student was also told that the cystostomy tube is only irrigated if absolutely necessary (*before* the drains are removed) because of the danger of increased bleeding.

When the student left the unit, one of the nurses continued to offer fluids to Mr. P., as well as to assist him with turning, coughing, and deep breathing, and to take his vital signs. These treatments were done on a 2-hour basis during the night so that longer rest periods would be afforded the patient. He was medicated twice for incisional pain. His dressing remained dry and intact, and the cystostomy tube was draining well.

The next morning the doctor removed the dressing and pulled the Penrose drains out of the prostatic bed. A scultetus binder was used to keep the new dressings in place; the tails were placed so as to *surround* the cystostomy tube and prevent its being compressed or kinked. The patient tolerated the treatment well. During the dressing change, the doctor explained to Mr. P. that his diet was to be increased gradually and, therefore, IV fluids would be ordered for the day to supplement oral intake. The following orders were written subsequently:

Follow present IV with 2,500 ml D₅W, then D/C IV and progress diet.

Since *warm liquids* seem to decrease the severity of bladder spasms—which are commonly experienced when the bladder musculature is incised or invaded by bacteria—warm tea and warm lemonade were offered to Mr. P. However, he was unable to retain them; he had an emesis of 200 ml clear fluids.

The student who was assigned to his care on this first postoperative day assisted Mr. P. out of bed and into a chair which had been previously placed close to the bed so that he would not have to walk to reach it. (The order OOB-in-chair for the first postoperative day of the suprapubic prostatectomy patient usually means just that; *walking is not to be encouraged* because bleeding may be increased by this activity.) Once in the chair, Mr. P. was encouraged to cough and deep-breathe. The position was particularly conducive to fostering optimum ventilation, and the student assisted the patient by lending support to the operative area. A table was then placed close to the patient and he was thereby able to wash his face and brush his teeth. He remained OOB for a 15-minute interval and tolerated this well. He continued to complain of an urge to void, however. It was explained that the site of the operation—the area around the urinary outlet—accounted for the feeling and that most such patients experienced it. He seemed relieved to know that his experience was not unique and/or a sign of complications. He was further reassured that the cystostomy tube was draining the urine from his bladder.

After Mr. P. had been assisted back into bed, he was allowed to rest a while before his vital signs were taken. They were stable and he remained afebrile. The cystostomy tube was draining well—the drainage still quite bloody in appearance with small clots noted—but he continued to have a moderate bloody discharge from the urethra. In the early afternoon before he was given his bath, the student carefully draped the patient; fan-folding the top sheet downward to expose the operative area while still affording cover for the pubic area to minimize embarrassment of the patient. After the soiled binder was opened and the wet dressings removed, the student elevated the cystostomy tube *gently* (so as not to initiate a bladder spasm) with one hand and began cleansing the urosanguinous drainage from the area immediately around the tube and adjacent to the incisional line before cleansing the intact skin of the area. (*Cleansing strokes should never be directed from the intact skin area toward the exposed tissue around the tube or toward the edges of the suture line* because skin bacteria may be swept into those areas, predisposing the patient to infection.) When the sterile dressings had been applied and a sterile towel placed over them to keep them in place, Mr. P. was asked to support the towel with his forearms and turn slightly toward one side so that the soiled binder could be removed and a clean one placed under him. He maintained the position for a short interval while the student washed his entire back region and inserted the clean binder. Subsequently, the dressings were secured in place with the binder and the patient's bath was completed. (*The binder was not wrapped firmly because its purpose was to secure the dressings and not to provide support for the area.*) He was afforded privacy while he washed the pubic and perineal region and was allowed to place the abdominal pads where they could absorb the bloody urethral discharge. The patient was medicated for pain, offered fluids thereafter and was allowed to rest.

The pathology report was received on the unit later in the afternoon. The prostatic parenchyma appeared nodular with large areas of cystic change and proliferation. The connective tissue in the other areas had increased, but no atypical areas were identified. Thus the diagnosis of benign prostatic hypertrophy was confirmed.

The IV fluids ordered were completely absorbed by late evening and the needle was removed from the vein because the patient was tolerating oral fluids in small amounts. His dressings continued to be changed as needed and ventilation exercises continued at regular intervals.

By the second postoperative day, Mr. P. was tolerating fluids well. He was assisted out of bed into a chair. Since he had orders for progressive ambulation, was allowed to walk a short distance. He complained of burning in the urethra at intervals. In the early afternoon the cystostomy tube stopped draining and the student realized that an irrigation would be necessary. Since a clot was the probable cause of the blockage, it would be necessary to irrigate under pressure to express the clot and clear the passageway. To minimize the possibility of initiating a bladder spasm, the student lowered the height of the head of the bed to place the patient in a more horizontal position. Then gently and slowly instilled about 60 ml of irrigating solution into the bladder by exerting pressure on the rubber bulb of the irrigating syringe with the thumb. With the syringe still positioned in the cystostomy tube, the pressure on the bulb was *slowly* released—allowing solution and clots to be suctioned into the syringe. The procedure was repeated once more and Mr. P. tolerated it well. The tube was patent and draining thereafter. Bladder spasms did increase in severity and frequency during that day and the doctor was notified. An antispasmodic table QID was ordered, and this seemed to diminish the severity of the spasms when they occurred. The student also advised the patient to try to take slow, deep breaths during those episodes so as to encourage generalized relaxation of the body. The dressings were changed frequently.

On the third postoperative day fewer dressing changes were needed and the drainage was pink-tinged. The bloody urethral drainage had subsided and, since they remained stable, the vital signs were ordered O.D. The patient was placed on a regular diet. Since his activity was being gradually progressed and the student realized that he would be fully ambulatory by the next day, Mr. P. was instructed regarding the transport of the drainage bag. He was told that it should always be carried *below* the level of the bladder and that urine should not be allowed to back up in the tubing. He was also shown how to manipulate the tubing so that urine trapped in it would flow into the collecting receptacle. During the course of the following day the student noted that Mr. P. always carried the drainage bag at arms length when walking. He hooked it to the lowermost part of the chair close to the floor when sitting (or it can be placed on the floor if drainage bottles in carrying baskets are used.)

The urine was amber-colored by the fourth postoperative day, except for one interval when bloody urine was noted in the tubing after the patient had gone to the bathroom and tried unsuccessfully to have a bowel movement. The student advised Mr. P. that his straining to force a bowel movement had caused pressure to be exerted on the operative area which was still healing. This had resulted in the bleeding episode. He was reassured that he had done no damage and that the bleeding would subside. He was then given a glass of *warm* prune juice—a half glass of prune juice with hot water added—to facilitate his next attempt. The doctor was notified and a suppository was ordered. Although the patient had a bowel movement subsequently and milk of magnesia 30 ml, H.S., PRN was allowed, daily requests for warm prune juice continued.

On the sixth postoperative day the combiotic was discontinued; and on the seventh postoperative day the patient was given 75 mg Demerol (IM) prior to the time that an 18 Fr Foley catheter with a 5-ml bag was inserted transurethrally. The catheter passed easily, and after it was successfully irrigated the cystostomy tube and all of the sutures were removed. The dressings were then frequently saturated with clear urine, necessitating many dressing changes. (The nursing staff did not pile on excessive layers of dressings to lengthen the intervals between dressing changes because they realized that this would only mean that urinary drainage would remain in contact with the patient's skin for prolonged periods and predispose Mr. P. to skin irritation.)

As the days passed, the suprapubic drainage diminished and the wound healed. When the wound was completely healed, the Foley catheter was removed and the patient kept a record of the time and amount of his voidings. Mr. P. continued to force fluids during this phase of his hospitalization. He did have complaints of "dribbling" of urine and urgency, so he was advised to urinate at regular intervals instead of waiting until the urge was overwhelming; he was also taught continence exercises (see Chapter 7). It was explained that the ringlike muscle (the sphincter) that helped him to control his urine was working sluggishly because of the tube that had been inserted through the penis, and that in a short time the muscle would regain its tone and begin working efficiently again. He followed the suggestions and the condition resolved itself.

Mr. P. was discharged on the morning of the fourteenth postoperative day. Before he left the unit, however, he was reminded not to do any heavy lifting or carrying for a month. He was told that he should anticipate occasional episodes of bleeding when voiding, but that the doctor should be notified if the amount or frequency increased. He was reminded that straining to force a bowel movement would tend to initiate bleeding. Mr. P. assured the nurse that he would take the mild laxative recommended by his doctor if he had any difficulty. When told that he should continue to drink about three quarts of fluid each day, he asked if there was an easy way that he could keep track of the amount he drank. He was advised that 12 to 14 glasses daily would fulfill the suggested quota. This information completed his preparation for discharge.

REFERENCES

1. Apfelback, G. L. Vas deferens reflux following prostatic surgery. J. Urol., 94:164–167, 1965.
2. Ashworth, A. Hydronephrosis. Practitioner, 197:605–610, 1966.
3. Badenoch, A. W. Benign enlargement of the prostate. Practitioner, 197:598–604, 1966.
4. Bruce, A. W., and Quirk, J. Prostatectomy and infection. J. Urol., 92:523–527, 1964.
5. Casteel, C. R., et al. Vas crush for prevention of post-prostatectomy epididymitis: An experimental and clinical study, J. Urol., 93:476–478, 1965.
6. Crassweller, P. O. Benign hyperplasia of the prostate. Canad. Nurse, 64:32–34, 1968.
7. Creevy, C. D. Reactions peculiar to transurethral resection of the prostate. Surg. Clin. N. Amer., 47:1471–1472, 1967.
8. Hall, A. Nursing care of patient following prostatectomy. Canad. Nurse, 64:35–37, 1968.
9. Haltiwanger, E. Management of benign prostatic hypertrophy. Surg. Clin. N. Amer., 45:1441–48, 1965.
10. Jameson, R. M., et al. Vasectomy and prostatectomy. Brit. J. Urol., 40:433–40, 1968.
11. Jordan, W. P., et al. Cryosurgery of the prostate: A preliminary report. J. Urol., 98:512–515, 1967.
12. Kasselman, M. J. Nursing care of the patient with benign prostatic hypertrophy. Amer. J. Nurs., 66:1026–30, 1966.
13. Marshall, A. Retropubic prostatectomy: A review with special

reference to urinary infection. Brit. J. Urol., 39:307–328, 1967.

14. Plorde, J. J., et al. Course and prognosis of prostatectomy. New Eng. J. Med., 272:269–277, 1965.

15. Ray, E. H. Bladder neck obstruction due to prostatic hyperplasia: Diagnosis, treatment and postoperative care. Amer. Surg., 31:325–328, 1965.

16. Roen, P. R. Atlas of Urologic Surgery. New York, Appleton-Century-Crofts, 1967.

17. Symposium on the problems of prostatic obstruction. Brit. J. Surg., 52:744–757, 1965.

18. Tuffill, S. G. Prostatic enlargement—its surgical and nursing treatment. Nurs. Mirror, 14:1–5, 11–12, 1964.

19. Wakeley, J. Urinary outflow obstruction in the male. Nurs. Mirror, 126:17–21, 1968.

20. Ward, R. J., et al. Respiratory function after transurethral resection. Dis. Chest, 49:298–301, 1966.

21. Sears, B. R. Benign prostatic obstruction. Med. Sci., 604–626, 1960.

7

The Patient with Cancer of the Prostate

Malignant tumors of the genitourinary tract are most frequently observed in the prostate gland, the bladder, and the kidney; carcinoma of the prostate is the most common type. Although not limited to men in the older age group, cancer of the prostate is found primarily in men over 55 years of age, and it ranks second to pulmonary malignancies as a cause of death in adult male patients.

As reviewed in the previous chapter, the prostate lies anterior to the rectum, surrounding the bladder neck and the proximal part of the urethra; its anterior surface faces the symphysis pubis. It is partly muscular, partly glandular, and is composed of four lobes which are encapsulated by a thin, firm membrane of smooth muscle and fibrous tissue. Of the four lobes—the posterior, two lateral, and the median—the posterior lobe of the gland is believed to be the site of origin of carcinoma. Early investigators thought that the lesion began as a tiny nodule on the posterior surface of the gland in the peripheral prostatic tissue close to the rectal wall, but current evidence indicates that it may begin as several distinct masses within various segments of the gland. Foci have been found in the periurethral portions of the prostate as well as in posterior prostatic tissue, but the incidence of indurated areas felt in posterior portions of the gland is greater.

The lesion may be identified during the patient's annual physical examination when a small, firm nodule in the posterior or lateral portions of the gland is felt on rectal palpation (see Fig. 1). It should be noted, however, that rectal examination alone cannot confirm a diagnosis of prostatic cancer: not all firm areas within the prostate are cancerous. Areas of developing benign hyperthrophy, or fibrosis, focal infection, calculi, infarctions, and/or tuberculous lesions may also produce such areas of induration. Therefore, a differential diagnosis must be made, and prostatic biopsy is always indicated.

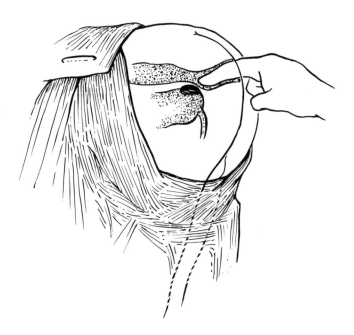

Fig. 1. The rectal examination. Note the proximity of the prostate gland to the rectal wall.

There are numerous theories as to the cause of prostatic cancer; the most popular ones include sexual excess, sexual decline, stagnation of prostatic secretions owing to loss of muscular tone in the gland, circulatory changes secondary to arteriosclerosis and venous thrombosis, and hormonal change that reflects the aging process. Moreover, none of these hypotheses has been adequately substantiated, and the etiology of prostatic cancer remains essentially unknown. It is known, however, that androgen administration tends to speed up the rate of growth of the carcinoma while estrogen administration tends to slow down the rate of growth. Therefore, it would seem that the best theory as to the etiology of prostatic cancer is that the condition reflects a disturbance in the circulating androgen-estrogen ratio in older men.

Early carcinoma of the prostate gland—localized within the capsule—does not produce symptoms. Commonly, the general health of the patient is good. This is the reason for the recommendation that men over 40 years of age should have a rectal examination included as part of their annual physical. By the time the patient begins to complain of the discomforts of lower urinary-tract obstruction (i.e., the symptoms of prostatism that were discussed in Chapter 6), the carcinoma has extended to the prostatic urethra and to the bladder neck. Hematuria usually occurs as a late manifestation when the bladder has been invaded. The presenting complaint may even be that of acute retention and/or infection. It should be remembered, therefore, that the patient with prostatic cancer usually remains asymptomatic until late in the course of the disease. The symptoms manifested are the result of local extension or metastasis of the carcinoma.

Characteristically, the tumor spreads from the prostate gland to the seminal vesicles, the bladder neck, and the lymph nodes of the pelvis. The fascia separating the prostate from the rectum seems to be resistant to prostatic carcinoma as infiltration into the rectum is rare. The tumor cells may spread from the regional pelvic lymph nodes to the nodes surrounding the aorta and to the inguinal lymph chain. From there, they may spread to the cervical and supraclavicular lymphatics. In addition to local infiltration and lymphatic extension, metastases via the bloodstream are common. This occurs by way of the vertebral veins, and usually affects the lumbar vertebrae, the pelvis, the ribs, and the femurs. Metastasis to the lungs and liver may also be accomplished by this route. If the tumor cells spread to the skeletal structure, the patient experiences deep, constant, severe pain. He may complain of pain in the lumbosacral region which radiates to the hips or down both legs. Extensive bony involvement may even predispose the patient to pathologic fractures. When there is bone marrow involvement, the weakness, weight loss, and eventual emaciation associated with anemia results. Such signs as peripheral edema—especially in the area of the scrotum and/or lower extremities—may be indicative of extensive regional involvement. This causes subtle but increasing pressure on the pelvic veins and lymphatics, resulting in their gradual occlusion. Extension of the tumor from the bladder neck or seminal vesicles to the area of the ureters may result in obstruction that leads to hydronephrosis. When this occurs, the patient may complain of flank pain. The prognosis is poor in this instance, and death often ensues.

DIAGNOSTIC PROCEDURES

Whatever the patient's presenting symptoms, the student should remember that nursing personnel will be in closest contact with the patient during the diagnostic period. Nothing will encourage the patient to adjust to his new surroundings more than a friendly, understanding, explanatory attitude. Such an approach or personal presentation will inspire trust and confidence and often facilitates the implementation of care during more crucial periods of the patient's hospitalization. Since these patients are usually elderly, an unhurried manner will often save time for the student. Elderly patients often balk when hurried, and the compliance sought will be delayed if care is attempted in an impatient or abrupt manner.

After the patient's admission, the diagnostic work-up usually includes blood work, renal-function tests, an electrocardiogram, cystoscopic examination, chest and skeletal x-ray series, and an IVP. The cardiogram aids in the assessment of the patient's general physical status, cystoscopy helps the urologist rule out associated bladder pathology, and the skeletal series confirms or rules out metastases. Open or closed perineal biopsy may also be indicated. Such a barrage of tests and treatments being imposed on an individual who may be experiencing his first hospitalization enhances the need for emotional support. Encouragement from members of the nursing team is an as invaluable adjunct to the medical plan.

Just as the rectal examination is essential for the *early diagnosis* of prostatic cancer, the serum acid phosphatase determination is important in the diagnosis of late, advanced lesions of the prostate. It is believed that this enzyme is involved in the breakdown of glucose into fructose, which serves as food for spermatozoa. Most of the acid phosphatase measured in the serum is produced by the blood cells, the liver, and the spleen. Under normal conditions, the quantities of this enzyme which are derived from the cells of the prostate are found in high concentration in prostatic secretions and also in the urine and seminal fluid. Prostatic acid phosphatase is present in the serum in minute amounts only. However, in the presence of advanced prostatic carcinoma when there is extensive metastasis, the serum acid phosphatase level may rise secondary to increased amounts of the enzyme being produced by the neoplastic cells and liberated into the circulating blood. The student should be aware that such an elevation may also occur subsequent to prostatic massage or manipulation and/or instrumentation of the prostatic portion of the urethra. Further, it should be noted that fever may cause depression of the serum acid phosphatase level. Although false elevations or depressions of this type are transient, blood for acid phosphatase determination should be drawn at least 24 hours *after* a rectal examination or cystoscopy, and the patient should be afebrile.

X-ray examination of the skeletal structure—including the pelvis, spine, and rib cage—is always an important diagnostic tool when prostatic carcinoma is suspected. The flat, marrow-bearing bones will reveal areas of increased density which resemble snowflakes. Such findings are of great value in the evaluation of advanced cases of prostatic cancer. Blood work will reveal an elevation in the *alkaline phosphatase* level when bony metastasis is present.

All of the procedures mentioned thus far are important diagnostic aids, but biopsy is the only procedure which will definitely establish the diagnosis of cancer of the prostate. Currently, two approaches are utilized frequently: the transrectal approach, and the perineal approach. The retropubic approach for biopsy allows for the inspection of the iliac lymph nodes, but—as the carcinomatous lesion usually occurs near the posterior surface of the prostate—the gland has to be elevated and rotated to allow visualization of the lesion. Therefore, the retropubic approach *for biopsy* is not done. When the transrectal approach is utilized, the colon is not usually prepared. (Urologists feel that it is not necessary to give Neomycin orally at regular intervals during the day prior to the procedure so that the possibility of infection will be reduced. Cleansing enemas are also omitted.) The perianal shave and scrub is usually completed immediately preceding biopsy. Thereafter, needle biopsy is achieved through the rectal wall (after a rectal examination serves to locate the area of induration). The biopsy needle is placed anterior to the examining finger, which acts as a position guide (see Fig. 2).

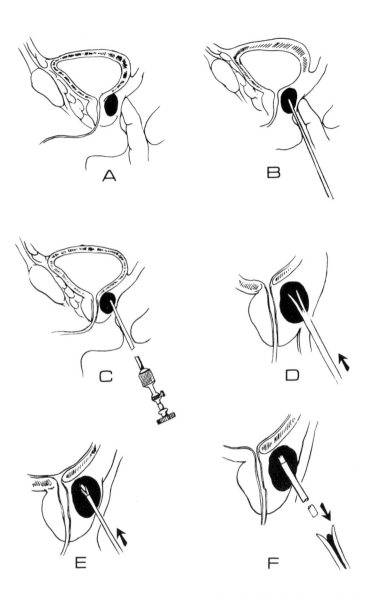

Fig. 2. Use of the biopsy needle. A. Nodule palpated with finger. B. Finger used as a guide to position needle. C. Pointed stylus replaced with flanged stylus. D. Flanged stylus advanced through shaft into nodule. E. Shaft advanced over flanges (note arrow). F. Flanges with biopsied tissue withdrawn through shaft. (From Scott, R. **J.A.M.A.**, 201:12, 1967. Courtesy of American Medical Association, and Dr. Russell Scott.)

The perineal needle biopsy is mechanically easy to perform; it may even be done on an out-patient basis. With the patient in lithotomy position and a finger of one hand of the examiner's inserted into the rectum to support the gland in the region of the lesion, the urologist introduces the biopsy needle through the perineum with his other hand. The patient who is found to have prostatitis, tuberculosis, or an infarction and not carcinoma may thus be spared the trauma of an open prostatic biopsy. The open perineal approach is more accurate, however, as it allows for direct visualization of the lesion and minimizes error in excision. It also permits radical surgery to be performed immediately if the frozen sections confirm the suspicion of malignancy.

Since there is a possibility that hemorrhage may occur from the urethra or bladder with extravasation into the retropubic space, vital signs should be taken at regular intervals following prostatic biopsy. The student should also note when (or if) the patient voids following biopsy, and the urine should be observed for blood. The nurse's notes should state whether hematuria was noted. If the patient becomes febrile, especially following transrectal biopsy, the doctor should be notified as antibiotic therapy may be indicated.

The student will usually find the patient quite apprehensive during this phase of the diagnostic work-up, but may feel uneasy about allowing him to voice his fears. It should be remembered, therefore, that most patients expect the nurse to be a good listener so that they may express their thoughts. Although the nurse may pose thought-evoking questions or healthful alternatives in certain situations, the comfort given in most instances is in the empathetic relationship which develops in the nurse-patient contact. Often a response such as "I can appreciate how you must feel" or "That must have been upsetting; I'll bet you're glad it's over with" is sufficient to make the patient feel better emotionally. In other words, it is the *sharing* of an experience that comforts. The nurse's feelings about cancer may also tend to color perception of the patient's viewpoint, and this should be considered during any interaction with a patient suspected of having cancer. Avoiding conversaiton with the patient only reinforces his feelings of dejection and alienation from others; and, in like manner, changing the subject during conversations when the patient wants to talk about his physical condition reinforces the belief that he is not being told the truth. *Ascertaining* what the patient has been told by his doctor, *assisting* him to focus on this, *clarifying* the things that may not have been understood, and *correcting* distortions of information previously given often prove encouraging to the patient.

METHODS OF TREATMENT

The choice of treatment for carcinoma of the prostate is made after the diagnostic work-up has been completed. If there is a positive tissue biopsy with the nodule confined within the prostatic capsule and if there is no evidence of metastases (i.e., findings of a normal serum acid phosphatase level and a negative x-ray series), the treatment of choice for carcinoma of the prostate is usually radical prostatectomy. Radical prostatectomy involves the removal of the entire prostate gland along with the seminal vesiculectomy and excision of the bladder neck—the remainder of the bladder then being anastamosed to the membranous urethra (see Fig. 3). Other considerations for this treatment approach are age and cardiopulmonary and renal status. If the patient is under 70 years of age and has a life expectancy of ten years or more, and if the patient has no significant limitations in the physical areas mentioned, radical surgery is recommended. A perineal or retropubic approach (see Fig. 4) may be utilized to accomplish

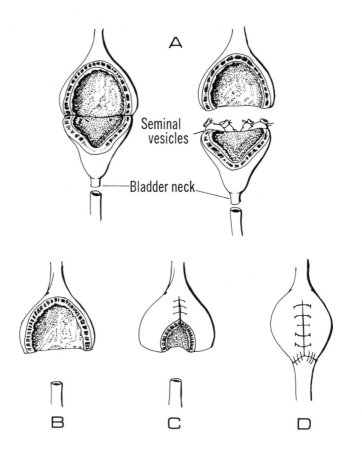

Fig. 3. Radical prostatectomy. A. The entire prostrate gland is excised. The seminal vesicles and bladder neck are excised along with the prostate. B, C, and D. The remainder of the bladder must be tapered so that it can be anastomosed to the membranous urethra.

this; and, since the ensuing postoperative problems are those of incontinence and impotence, the doctor usually discusses these eventualities with the patient.

It is usually explained that many patients exhibit varying degrees of incontinence: from the stress incontinence that follows coughing or straining to the total incontinence which

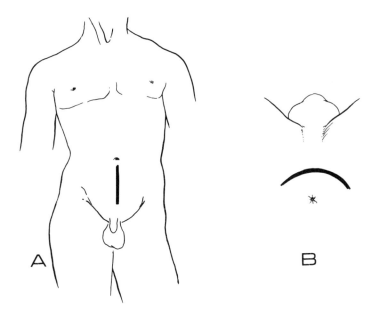

Fig. 4. A. Incisional site for the radical retropubic prostatectomy. B. Incisional site for the radical perineal prostatectomy. The nurse should remember that the perineum is located behind the scrotum and in front of the anus.

necessitates the use of a urinary drainage apparatus. During the first three postoperative months, some degree of incontinence may be expected; however, urinary control through sphincter exercise may be regained within the first six months of the postoperative period. The internal sphincter includes the area of the bladder neck and adjacent areas of the prostatic urethra. This structure is removed during radical prostatectomy and, therefore, cannot function in urinary control. Thus intraurethral resistance to the outflow of urine must be developed to effect urinary continence. The external sphincter, levator ani, and perineal muscles exert an effect on the membranous urethra —which is sufficient to control urination. They increase tension on its walls, thereby decreasing the lumen of that area of the urethra. It is therefore understandable how exercise of the sphincter and muscles mentioned will help the patient to regain continence. If the patient is employed, he may have serious reservations about the operation because the possibility of incontinence may necessitate a change of occupation. The nurse should allow the patient to express these considerations because such a change at this stage of his life is usually crucial. Once again, the good listener may provide the emotional support needed.

Teaching *prior to operation* will make it easier for the patient to master the method by which continence exercise may be accomplished. The student may thus provide an invaluable service to the patient. Active exercise consists of the repeated contraction of rectal and urethral sphincters. The patient should be instructed to refrain from concurrently tensing the musculature of his abdominal wall. He should also be told that he should be able to observe penile retraction during the exercise. It is this retraction which may serve as an index of his ability to execute the exercise properly. In many cases prostatic obstruction results in sluggish functioning of the external sphincter secondary to disuse; it should be explained that active, conscientious effort must be expended to achieve continence after surgical intervention.

Following radical prostatectomy the patient is usually impotent because of the removal of the periprostatic nerve supply. However, the question of retained potency in patients of this age group is often of little significance. It should be remembered that alternative hormonal therapy—estrogen administration subsequent to castration—is likely to present the same problem.

Of the two approaches available, the radical perineal prostatectomy is more frequently performed. Although the retropubic approach is preferred when the gland is large and situated high in the pelvic cavity, considerable difficulty in anastomosing the bladder to the urethra may be encountered.

Complications may occur in the postoperative period because of inefficient wound drainage. Also a candidate for the retropubic approach would be a debilitated patient or one who had significant cardiac, respiratory, or renal limitations. Such a patient could not withstand an extended period of time in the exaggerated lithotomy position necessary for the perineal approach.

With the perineal approach, prolonged perineal drainage is usually the primary factor in extended hospitalization. Epididymitis may occur in many instances even when the vas deferens is ligated deep in the pelvis. However, it has been found that the occurrence of epididymitis diminishes when *scrotal* vasectomy is performed (Culp, 1967).

POSTOPERATIVE CARE

In the immediate recovery period the vital signs are usually taken every 15 minutes until they are stable. Thereafter, they may be taken hourly for 4 hours and then every 2 hours for a 24-hour period. The patient must be afforded rest during the first postoperative night; thus the patient's turning, deep breathing, and coughing should be encouraged at intervals that coincide with the taking of his vital signs. The student should always remember to take the vital signs *prior to* assisting the patient with the aforementioned activities. Vigorous coughing should be avoided, but adequate deep breathing and movement must be insured (unless specifically contraindicated by doctor's orders) if respiratory complications are to be avoided. It must also be remembered that *the patient should be medicated for pain* if he is to be expected to accomplish those postoperative tasks which are so vital to his survival. A patient cannot be expected to turn, cough, or deep-breathe in the first 48 postoperative hours without medication for pain. Further, the fact that medication is not requested will not be an acceptable excuse for failing to administer it—*especially*

when it is observed that the patient refuses to cooperate. Mos
patients abhor injections, and many older patients will lie sti
—restricting movement so as to avoid pain—rather than as
for medication or "bother the busy nurse who has so man
others to care for." The patient should be encouraged to coug
and deep-breathe every hour during the daytime hours of th
first two postoperative days. Some urologists will order a pos
itive-pressure breathing apparatus as a prophylactic measur
to insure proper lung expansion and to prevent atelectasis. Thi
therapy may be extended until x-ray examination confirms tha
the lungs are clear; it is well known that older patients ar
predisposed to respiratory complications. An elevation in tem
perature is often indicative of the accumulation of mucus in th
lungs and should serve as a warning to the nurse that th
patient is not coughing effectively. Oral temperatures ar
usually taken because the surgical area is in such close prox
imity to the rectum that the danger of trauma to the site o
anastomosis is present.

If the surgical procedure has been accomplished throug
a retropubic approach, drains will usually be placed on eithe
side of the bladder and deep in the pelvis. The patient wil
always have a urethral catheter in place; this serves a dua
function: to effect urinary drainage and to splint the ure
throvesical anastomosis. A cystostomy tube may also be pres
ent. The Foley catheter in the urethra usually remains in plac
—without being changed—for approximately 2 weeks or unti
complete healing occurs, and the doctor will usually order PRN
irrigations. These irrigations should be done only when th
catheter begins to drain sluggishly and *not routinely* during
each tour of duty. If gentle irrigation is unsuccessful in clear
ing the lumen of the catheter, the doctor should be notified and
another catheter of like dimension should be available on th
unit for his use if a change is necessary. To prevent traction
on the urethral catheter, it should be taped to the inner aspec
of the thigh (as indicated in Chapter 3, Fig. 2a, p. 42).

Because of the possibility of paralytic ileus, postoperative oral intake is usually restricted until bowel sounds are audible. The patient is then often placed on a liquid diet in the early postoperative period and the kind and amount of food allowed is gradually increased according to the patient's progress. Daily weighings are usually ordered—the patient being weighed in the mornings before breakfast—and the accuracy of these must be stressed because weight gain can be an index of fluid retention. Accurate intake *and* output is essential at this stage of the patient's postoperative course. Total intake should include the enumeration of both oral and IV intake. In situations in which fluids are given by clysis, the amount of fluid absorbed must also be included. When the patient is able to tolerate solid foods, the student may find that only small amounts are eaten at each meal. Supplementary feedings are often indicated in such instances and the patient should be encouraged to eat small amounts frequently. The student should check to insure that the tray presented has an uncluttered look. This may be accomplished by removing some parts of the meal and storing them in the refrigerator so that they may be given as between-meal supplementary feedings. If the patient has to be assisted at mealtime, he should not be rushed. Rather than have the food "shoveled" into his mouth, the patient will insist after a few mouthfuls that he has had enough or that he is not hungry.

Total output should include urinary drainage (as well as vomitus and gastric-suction returns if applicable). An approximation of the amount of drainage present on dressings during the day should also be indicated. Usually the dressings may be changed PRN and, when dressing changes are recorded on the nurses' notes, the amount and color of the drainage present on the soiled dressing should be noted. However, an approximation of the total amount of such drainage is often missing from the summary sheet of the patient's daily progress. It must be remembered that this drainage is also representative of output. Such inclusion is usually indicated by the plus sign (+): 1+

denoting a scant to small amount of drainage present on dressings, 2+ denoting a moderate to large amount of drainage, and 3+ denoting saturated dressings.

Elastic bandages are often ordered for the patient following radical prostatectomy. These are usually to be wrapped from the toes to the groin region, and the student should not leave the heel exposed. The bandages should be reapplied daily, and the student will often find that this can be done at the time the bath is given. If the elastic bandages are removed *before* the bath is given, opportunity is afforded for the washing of the patient's legs and feet. Owing to the loss of some of the skin turgor because of aging, it will be noted upon removal that the bandages—however carefully applied—leave ridges in the patient's skin. Breakdown areas will tend to develop if the bandages are not removed to allow for a release of the pressure on the legs. Usually these ridges will be seen to disappear during the course of the bath, and the student may observe the condition of the skin in those otherwise-covered areas at this time.

Ambulation begins early in the patient's postoperative course—often as early as the first postoperative day—and the patient should be encouraged to increase his out-of-bed activity progressively. Patients may anticipate a postoperative hospital stay of approximately four weeks if the retropubic approach has been utilized; with the perineal approach, a three-week postoperative stay is average. However, because of the relatively slow recovery process and worries about the urinary "dribbling" that will be experienced when the urethral catheter is removed, patients often become dejected. The student should therefore encourage the patient to resume practice of the continence exercises taught in the preoperative period. These may be started as early as the third postoperative day, and the patient should continue them for the remainder of his convalescence. It must be remembered that the use of supportive urinary devices such as clamps, pads, or a condom-drainage apparatus are to be discouraged. They tend to decrease the motivation to strive for voluntary urinary control. It is therefore during the interval *before* the urethral catheter is removed that the patient should practice the perineal exercises so that urinary control may be regained more uneventfully after the removal of the Foley. When the patient begins to void, he should be told that he can voluntarily stop the urinary stream by tensing his perineal muscles. He should then be instructed to practice starting and stopping the stream several times a day, and he should be reassured that no artificial device can take the place of sphincter action. Worries about incontinence may be verbalized again immediately prior to discharge—the patient and/or his relatives may be particularly concerned about this situation in relation to his ability to enjoy activities away from home. In some cases the doctor may prescribe a urinary collecting apparatus, but both patient and family should be reminded that it may take a long time for continence to be regained and it should be emphasized that the exercises should be continued.

When the carcinoma has spread through the prostatic capsule, radical surgery is not the treatment of choice. The cancer is no longer curable at this stage and treatment is geared primarily toward palliation. Bilateral orchidectomy (removal of the testes, or castration) and administration of estrogen accomplish this goal. It is known that the growth of prostatic cancer is dependent upon the androgenic hormone. Therefore, with the removal of the testes, the primary source of that hormone is taken away and there is a decrease in the rate of growth of the carcinoma. Further, it is believed that the androgenic activity of the testes is dependent upon the effect of FSH (follicle-stimulating hormone). Since estrogen has a direct inhibitory effect on FSH production (estrogen → ↓ FSH production), it will have an indirect inhibitory effect on androgenic hormone production from the secondary or extragonadal sources once bilateral orchidectomy has been performed. (Estrogen → ↓ FSH production → ↓ androgenic hormone production.) Some investigators believe that estrogens exert a depressive effect upon the prostatic cancer cells. Usually, estrogen is administered in the form of stilbestrol in doses of from 5 to 10 mg (po) TID.

The localized, painful, metastatic lesion in the vertebrae, hips, or long bones may be the chief complaint of a patient with prostatic carcinoma. Most of these patients respond favorably to hormonal therapy. Orchidectomy and/or estrogen therapy—while they may not markedly lengthen the lifespan of the average patient with metastatic cancer of the prostate—do provide relief from pain. The student will also usually notice an improvement in the appetite and outlook of the patient.

For patients in which the lesions remain painful in spite of hormonal therapy or for those who experience a relapse from hormonal control, radiotherapy is frequently instituted. Although the prostatic cancer cells tend to be relatively radioresistant, adequate dosage may produce regression of the lesion. Deep x-ray treatment used to be restricted to areas of bony metastases. Currently, radiotherapy is being used as definitive primary treatment rather than for palliation. The injection of radioactive gold directly into the prostatic tumor has also been utilized. Since the radiation from this isotope consists of short, penetrating beta rays and the half-life is only 65 hours, undesirable radiation of surrounding structures can be avoided. Also, radioactive phosphate may be given intravenously. It seems to concentrate primarily in the bony metastatic lesions, where its beta rays effect their influence without harming blood-forming tissue. The student will observe that estrogen administration is discontinued and testosterone therapy begun when radioactive phosphate is given. This is done to encourage increased uptake of the radioactive phosphate. Pain is usually relieved shortly after such therapy is instituted and the patient feels he has improved.

Other palliative measures include transurethral resection (TUR) when vesical outlet obstruction causes retention, or suprapubic cystostomy if a TUR cannot be performed and urinary drainage is seriously compromised. In these instances, the patient's comfort is especially important; the nurse should endeavor to insure good diet, plenty of rest, and rapport at all times. Recurrence of the cancerous lesion in the membranous urethra may cause the urologist to resort to adrenalectomy as a palliative measure. It is believed that adrenal androgens may also stimulate the growth of the prostatic cancer cells; thus, the removal of these glands should tend to inhibit their growth. Hypophysectomy has been performed for patients in relapse after castration-estrogen therapy. It is believed that the pituitary gland may have something to do with neoplastic growth because of the action of its growth hormone, and hypophysectomy may act to inhibit certain forms of malignant tumors.

REFERENCES

1. Culp, O. S. Radical perineal prostatectomy: Its past, present, and possible future. J. Urol., 98:618–626, 1967.
2. Flint, L. D., et. al. Radical prostatectomy for carcinoma of the prostate. Surg. Clin. N. Amer., 47:695–705, 1967.
3. Jewett, H. J. Treatment of early cancer of the prostate. J.A.M.A., 183:373–375, 1963.
4. Jorgens, J. The radiographic characteristics of carcinoma of the prostate. Surg. Clin. N. Amer., 45:1427–1439, 1965.
5. Lattimer, J. K. Prostatic carcinoma—Number one cancer in older men. Sem. Rep., 2:2–8, 1957.
6. Lilien, O. M., et al. The case for perineal prostatectomy. J. Urol., 99:79–86, 1968.
7. Mellinger, G. T. Carcinoma of the prostate. Surg. Clin. N. Amer., 45:1413–1426, 1965.
8. Millard, O. H. Carcinoma of the prostate. Nova Scotia Med. Bull., 46:51–53, 1967.
9. Mossholder, I. B. When the patient has a radical retropubic prostatectomy. Amer. J. Nurs., 62:101–104, 1962.
10. Samellas, W. Urinary control following radical perineal prostatectomy. J. Urol., 95:580–583, 1966.

11. Scott, R. Needle biopsy in carcinoma of the prostate. J.A.M.A., 201:958–960, 1967.
12. Scott, W. W., and Toole, W. N. Carcinoma of the prostate. In Campbell, M. F., ed. Urology, 2nd ed. Philadelphia, W. B. Saunders Company, pp. 1173–1226, 1963.

8

The Patient with Cancer of the Testicle

Tumors of the testicle are comparatively rare, but most of them are malignant, and mortality is high. Bilateral testicular involvement is seldom seen. In contrast, although tumors of the epididymis and spermatic cord are also rare, they are usually benign. Cancer of the testicles is a disease of young men; it occurs primarily between the ages of 20 and 35, during the years of greatest sexual activity. Black and Oriental males are seldom afflicted. Most civilian hospital staffs encounter patients with this disease infrequently; however, because of the concentration of large numbers of young men in the armed forces, military hospitals are likely to have a number of patients present for treatment and care.

Tumors of the testicle are named for the type of tissue which predominates. Accordingly, they may be grouped into two general categories: those that can be classified as germinal tumors and those that can be classified as nongerminal tumors. For the purpose of this text, it will suffice to say that the germinal tumors include the pure seminoma, embryonal carcinoma (adenocarcinoma), teratoma, and choriocarcinoma; the nongerminal tumors include Leydig cell tumors, testicular adenomas (androblastomas), lymphomas, reticulum cell sarcomas, and other types of metastatic tumors. Pure seminomas are of relatively low malignancy, but they account for less than half of the germinal tumors. In the disease, testicular tissue is usually replaced with a firm tumorous mass that remains encapsulated. About a third of the malignant germinal tumors are adenocarcinomas, which tend to replace only part of the testicle but extend beyond the capsule. Hemorrhaging within the tumor often occurs (see Fig. 1). Teratomas com-

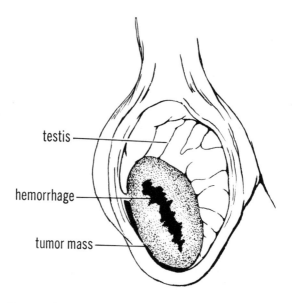

Fig. 1. Tumors of the testes. Note the area of hemorrhage within the tumor mass.

prise only a small percentage of germinal tumors and seldom extend beyond the testicular capsule. Only ½ to 1 percent of germinal tumors are choriocarcinomas, and they are usually fatal. Since they tend to be small in size, local signs of a hard testicular mass are often absent and the patient is frequently found to have metastatic lesions during the course of the diagnostic work-up.

The etiology of cancer of the testicle is essentially unknown, but evidence indicates that there is a higher incidence in atrophic gonads. Whether atrophy is secondary to cryptorchidism (undescended testicle), orchitis (inflammation of the testicle), or congenital abnormality, it is believed that a degenerative process within the testicle—related to some primary germ cell defect—may initiate malignant changes. Normally, fetal testes descend from the peritoneal cavity through the inguinal canal and are located in the scrotum at birth; the majority descend into the scrotum by the eighth fetal month (see Fig. 2). However, a small percentage will remain in an abnormal location, and this condition is known as *cryptorchidism* (undescended or "hidden" testicle). Fortunately, unilateral cryptorchidism occurs more frequently than the bilateral condition. In the majority of cases, underlying endocrine abnormality is absent, and the operation of *orchiopexy* must be performed to position the undescended testis in the scrotum. Since it has been observed that the tissue in an undescended testicle seldom reaches functional maturity, orchiopexy is done to encourage normal spermatogenesis. However, even when successful orchiopexy has been performed, approximately half of the repositioned testes eventually lose their ability to form spermatozoa. It is unknown whether this condition results from testicular dysgenesis (faulty testicular development) occurring secondary to congenitally defective germinal tissue. It is believed, however, that retention of a testis in the abdominal cavity or inguinal region where the body temperature is higher than in the scrotum and where mechanical trauma is likely to occur may predispose the undescended testis to undergo degenerative changes. Clinical evidence reveals that these progressive degenerative changes begin about the age of six, and gradual involution of the gonad may be noted after

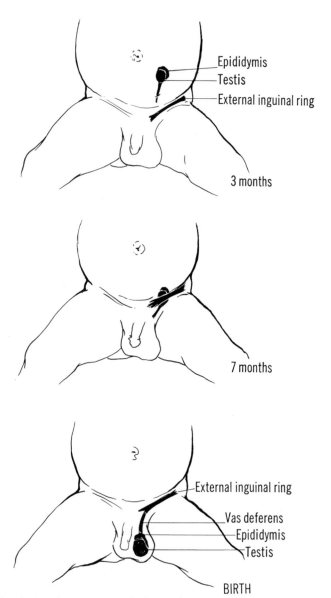

Fig. 2. Descent of the testes. The testes begin to descend from the peritoneal cavity at about the third month of fetal life. They traverse the inguinal canal by about the seventh month and usually descend into the scrotum (where they are located at birth) by the eighth fetal month.

198

this time. Some authorities, therefore, advocate orchiopexy during the preschool years to insure optimal functioning of the undescended testis. Delay beyond the age of nine years—especially after the onset of puberty—is particularly undesirable as studies reveal a higher incidence of cancer of the testicle among patients who have undergone orchiopexy for cryptorchidism after age six.

Most malignant tumors of the testicle metastasize through lymphatic channels, although there are instances in which metastasis occurs through both the lymphatic and vascular systems. The lymphatic route is most common in seminomas, whereas blood-borne metastasis is the major route in teratocarcinomatous lesions. In descending chronology, lymphatic drainage of the testes includes nodes above the renal pedicles, nodes along the medial border of each kidney and upper ureter, periaortic lymph nodes extending to the level of the bifurcation of that vessel, and lymphatic chains along the common iliacs (see Fig. 3). This type of cancer tends to metastasize early to distant areas; and, although almost any structure of the body may be invaded, the primary site of metastasis is to the retroperitoneal lymph nodes, the cells being transported via lymphatic invasion. Involvement of the inguinal nodes is rare unless the scrotum is invaded. Metastasis via the bloodstream usually leads to involvement of the lungs, liver, kidneys, and occasionally bone and brain tissue.

The signs and symptoms manifested by the patient with cancer of the testicle are dependent upon the amount of local testicular involvement and the degree of metastatic spread. The testis may remain normal in size and shape, it may be diffusely involved and enlarged, or there may be a palpable nodular surface (see Fig. 4). Frequently, the patient will complain of a feeling of increased weight in the scrotum, and compression of the involved testis fails to elicit the pain characteristically manifested when a normal or inflamed testis is compressed. Although the classic sign of testicular tumor is

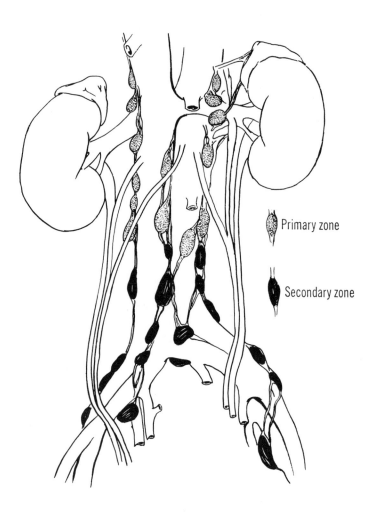

Fig. 3. Primary and secondary zones of lymph node involvement by testicular tumor. Included within the primary zone are the lymph nodes around the renal pedicle, the origin of the spermatic artery, and the insertion of the spermatic vein. The secondary zone includes the lateral aortic and iliac nodes. It should be noted, however, that at times the lateral aortic and iliac nodes may be the primary sites of metastasis. (From Kaufman, J. J. **Ca.** 17:55, 1967. Courtesy of Dr. Joseph Kaufman, and The American Cancer Society, Inc.)

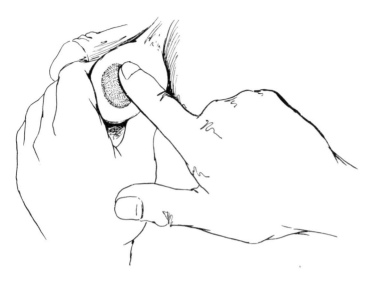

Fig. 4. Palpable nodular surface in the testis. In young adults, any lesion of the scrotum should be considered a tumor mass until evidence to the contrary is provided.

a *painless* hard and nodular mass in the testis, it should be noted that a large percentage of patients present with painful scrotal swellings and/or other symptoms (fever, nausea and vomiting, local heat, and skin redness) usually associated with an acute inflammation of the testis or epididymis. Unlike inflammatory processes, however, the varying degrees of pain experienced by these patients is often secondary to the weight of the tumor mass (see Fig. 5), hemorrhage within the tumor, or distention of the tunica albuginea caused by the tumorous growth. Further, the pain is usually *not relieved* by elevation of the scrotum. Urologists are usually alerted to the possibility of testicular tumor if the patient is young, complains of hardness and heaviness in the scrotum, reports a negative history of urinary or respiratory infection, and has a negative urinalysis and prostate examination. If palpation reveals a nodular or indurated area in the testis, a tumor is definitely suspect. The

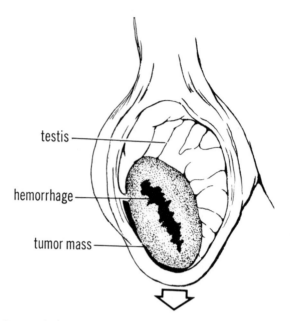

Fig. 5. Tumor of the testis. The arrow indicates the weight of the tumor, which tends to produce a feeling of increased weight in the scrotum. Varying degrees of pain may be experienced because of this weight, because of hemorrhage within the tumor, or because of distention of the tunica albuginea secondary to the growth of the tumor.

scrotum *does not transilluminate* unless a hydrocele has developed secondary to the tumor formation. Pain in the abdomen or the appearance of abdominal masses may also prompt the patient to seek medical advice; and, as the disease progresses, a chronic cough, appreciable weight loss and weakness, supraclavicular lymph node enlargement, and/or hepatomegaly may also be present.

Biopsy is seldom included in the diagnostic work-up of these patients because—owing to the threat of metastasis if it has not already occurred—care must be taken to avoid dispersion of the tumor cells. Since a unique feature of some of the malignant tumors of the testicle is the tendency to form chorionic gonadotrophins, determination of the presence of this hormone in the urine should be made. The student may remember that gonadotropins are normally manufactured by the anterior lobe of the pituitary and also by the chorionic villi of pregnant women. Thus the Aschheim-Zondek technique is the usual test employed to determine the presence of urinary chorionic gonadotropins; although a pregnancy determinant, the test is of diagnostic value for the male patient when testicular carcinoma is suspect. The student should collect the first-voided morning urine specimen and send it to the laboratory. Since these hormones are not formed by all of the malignancies, a negative test will not completely rule out the possibility of testicular tumor.

X-ray evidence is also taken into consideration. Evidence of metastases may be visible in chest films; intravenous urography may be invaluable because deviation of the ureters or outward displacement of the kidneys tend to signify retroperitoneal lymph-node involvement. Vena cavagrams aid in the diagnosis of retroperitoneal metastasis because enlargement of the lymph nodes in that area tends to cause displacement and/or compression of the vena cava. Currently, lymphangiography is also available. It is of value in the diagnosis of retroperitoneal lymph-node metastases and in the evaluation of the thoroughness of retroperitoneal lymph-node dissection.

TREATMENT MODALITIES

The treatment of malignant testicular tumors usually begins with radical orchiectomy, which is accomplished through an inguinal incision that resembles the type made for a classic herniorrhaphy. This approach permits high ligation of the spermatic cord so that exploration may guide the course of further treatment. After the diagnosis of tumor has been confirmed, the testis and that entire segment of the spermatic cord lying within the inguinal canal is removed. Then the peritoneum is opened just widely enough to allow the surgeon's hand to enter the peritoneal cavity so that lymph nodes along the vena cava and aorta may be palpated. Such exploration facilitates evaluation of the resectability of enlarged nodes, the eligibility of the patient for radical retroperitoneal lymphadenectomy, and/or the identification of the area toward which subsequent radiation therapy should be directed.

The type of tumor encountered during orchiectomy will dictate the course that additional treatment should take. Since the pure seminoma is so highly radiosensitive, a course of radiation therapy to the area of the regional lymphatics normally follows orchiectomy and urologists seldom advocate radical retroperitoneal lymph-node dissection. Conventional radiation dosages are usually directed to the iliac, umbilical, epigastric, lumbar, and lower dorsal regions. On the other hand, adenocarcinomas (embryonal carcinomas) and teratomas tend to be radioresistant and retroperitoneal lymph-node dissection is the preferred treatment. Additional treatment of pure choriocarcinomas is often thought to be fruitless since the course of the disease is seldom altered, and it is usually fatal. Metastasis usually occurs early via the bloodstream, and patients characteristically present complaining of symptoms of pulmonary and/or other distant metastatic lesions. Thus the disease is advanced by the time the patient seeks medical advice.

Radical surgery is generally accepted as the treatment of choice for those patients with extensive metastases. This type of surgical intervention usually includes the removal of distant metastatic lesions if they appear to be operable, and a series of operative procedures may be necessary: for example, orchiectomy, bilateral transperitoneal negative lymphadenectomy, and either segmental resection of pulmonary metastases or pneumonectomy. If *negative* retroperitoneal lymphadenectomy is performed, radiotherapy is often unnecessary.* However, if there

---

* Negative lymphadenectomy is the removal of lymph nodes which demonstrate no evidence of metastatic involvement; it is performed as a prophylactic measure to interrupt lymphatic routes which are likely to be invaded by testicular tumor cells.

is lymph-node involvement, radical surgery is usually followed by high-voltage radiation therapy.

During radiation therapy, the *observation* of the general health of the patient is an important nursing responsibility. Transfusions may be ordered if the signs of bone-marrow depression are present—if the white blood cell count is significantly altered or if anemia is revealed—and the student should always observe for untoward reactions at these times. The patient may complain of gastrointestinal distress and will often appear in acute distress during this phase of his postoperative course. If the patient's discomfort is *effectively* communicated to the doctor through *concise, accurate, pertinent* reporting, the nurse will be able to mobilize supportive measures that will sustain the patient and minimize symptoms during these postradiation intervals of acute illness.

There are several approaches which may be utilized to accomplish lymphadenectomy: the lumbar approach, the thoracolumbar approach, the transperitoneal approach, and the transabdominal approach. There is usually no impotence following the procedure because the dissection seldom involves pelvic structures. The operative approach usually determines the kind of care plan which the nursing staff should develop. If there is involvement of the thoracic cavity, the student will find that the care will be similar to that given a patient following chest surgery. If a lumbar incision is made, care will be similar to that given the patient with the flank incision (as discussed in Chapter 5); if the transabdominal route is taken, the care pertinent for the patient following abdominal operations is applicable. Observation for signs and symptoms of hemorrhage is of utmost importance since extensive stripping of the nodes along great vessels is involved during lymphadenectomy. The student will also remember that—although appropriate modifications may be necessary—principles of surgical nursing are applicable whenever an operation is performed, *regardless of the area of specialization* that is involved.

As for the other treatment modalities currently being

utilized for the care of a patient with testicular tumor, chemotherapeutic agents are under increasing investigation. Antibiotics and antimetabolites have been used with varying success, but data reflecting their use in the palliation of recurrent and advanced cases of testicular carcinoma are encouraging. Nitrogen mustard acts to slow the progression of the tumor, but its use has produced no cures. Most recent is the use of *triple drug therapy* which combines the effects of three of the most effective drugs: actinomycin D, chlorambucil, and methotrexate. These drugs are often given in conjunction with oral Furacin or nitrogen mustard; but they tend to be cytotoxic, with untoward side effects of severe leukopenia, diarrhea, stomatitis, or thrombocytopenia—which may cause the patient extreme discomfort. When given, the regimen usually consists of actinomycin D administered intravenously in five-day courses while concurrent daily dosages of oral chlorambucil and methotrexate are given. All three drugs are usually cancelled after the 25th day of the regimen, and maintenance therapy is given at regular (or irregular) intervals thereafter, according to the patient's progress.

In summary, the treatment modalities currently utilized in the management of tumors of the testicle include orchiectomy with high ligation of the spermatic cord, bilateral lymphadenectomy, irradiation of areas of metastatic spread, and chemotherapy. Radical surgery followed by radiotherapy and/or chemotherapy has resulted in increased percentages of five-year survivals even when patients have had metastatic lesions. Therefore, urologists feel justified in advocating an aggressive approach for the treatment of testicular tumors.

A NURSING-CARE STUDY

The student will find that little physical nursing care will be required by the patient with carcinoma of the testicle unless radical procedures are performed following orchiectomy. Except for postoperative discomfort (which is short-lived) and the symptoms of radiation sickness, these patients rarely suffer prolonged periods of acute physical distress during the course of their hospitalization. But continuous apprehension regarding any tests, procedures, and treatments performed during the preoperative and postoperative periods, as well as fear concerning the outcome of the pathology findings, tend to keep these patients in an *emotional* turmoil throughout their hospitalization. The patient will seldom verbalize these feelings to the student, but he will certainly experience severe postoperative dejection unless given adequate emotional support during his hospital stay. The nurse's role in the care of such a patient, therefore, is best illustrated by discussion of a particular case.

The patient, Mr. T., was a 24-year-old single, white male in no apparent distress; while admitting him to the unit the nurse discovered that this was his first hospitalization. He stated that he had been "swollen and hard down there" and was being admitted for surgery. After orienting Mr. T. to the unit (pointing out the bathroom, how to use the "call buzzer" to summon the nurse, the patients' recreation area, etc.), the nurse observed that he seemed to be nervous and uneasy. Before leaving, therefore, she introduced him to two of the younger patients on the unit so that he would be afforded the opportunity for diversional activity, and the three engaged in lively conversation.

The attending physician's note was then reviewed by the nurse, and she discovered that the patient had been told several years before that he had a hydrocele. However, during a recent physical examination, the left testicle was noted to be large and hard—four times the size of the right, and stony hard. As for pain, hematuria, discharge, and venereal disease, his report was negative. Admission had been advised for excision of the testicle to rule out malignancy. An IVP was to be part of the diagnostic work-up so that any ureteral deviation secondary to periaortic adenopathy could be demonstrated. After reviewing the note, the nurse notified the resident physician of the admission so that a history and physical could be done.

When the patient had been examined, the doctor wrote the following orders:

> Diet as tolerated
> Up ad lib
> CBC, urinalysis, serology, BUN, FBS
> Urine to lab for pregnancy test
> IVP and chest film tomorrow

The laboratory and x-ray slips were sent, and the patient was given a specimen bottle so that the required admission urinalysis could be obtained. At 7 P.M. that evening Mr. T. was told about the x-ray (IVP) he would have the next day, and it was explained that permission would have to be signed. He was given a cathartic, and seemed to understand the nurse's explanation of the rationale for this medication prior to IVP. Later that evening the patient was observed sitting alone in the solarium. The nurse spoke to him for a few moments, instructing him to take no liquids or food by mouth after midnight as the last part of his preparation for the x-ray, and he was also told that another urine specimen—his first urination of the morning—was needed for a special test that would provide information about the type of tissue causing the hardness of his testicle. A specimen bottle labeled with the patient's name had been left on his bedside table for his convenience and *as a reminder*. It was further explained to him that blood would be drawn in the morning as an aid in determining his overall physical condition; Mr. T. assured the nurse that he had always been in good health. They chatted a while about his parents and the family, and his work, and soon he seemed more relaxed and went to bed.

The next morning, the specimen for pregnancy

test was collected and sent to the laboratory. Later, on the way to the x-ray department, when the patient seemed tense, the nurse explained again what would be done during the IVP. The explanation and reassurance seemed to allay his apprehension. Good visualization of the abdomen was afforded by a scout film taken during the IVP; no evidence of metastatic lesions was revealed. Both kidneys were normal in size and shape, and the collecting systems (kidney pelvis, ureters, and bladder) were within normal limits. (This is referred to as a *negative IVP*—that is, without evidence of retroperitoneal mass.) A chest film was also taken, which revealed no abnormality; the lungs were clear, without evidence of metastatic lesion. Later that day, the doctor informed the patient that the "x-rays were good" and Mr. T. was greatly relieved. The nurse reinforced the patient's optimism by agreeing that the test results were good, and allowed him time to relate his conversation with the doctor. Fluids were forced during the rest of the day to make up for the period of dehydration prior to intravenous pyelography.

That evening, the nurse carried out the following orders:

> For left inguinal orchiectomy in A.M.
> Permission
> Shave and prep as for herniorrhaphy
> NPO after midnight
> Seconal 200 mg h.s.
> Seconal 200 mg at 11 A.M. tomorrow
> Demerol 50 mg ⎫ IM on call to OR
> Scopolamine 0.4 mg ⎭

After ascertaining that the patient understood the operative procedure that was to be done, the nurse witnessed the signing of the operative permit. The patient was shaved appropriately and instructed to wash the area with an antibacterial soap which the nurse provided. That evening, before giving the patient sleeping medication, the nurse told him to take nothing by mouth after the medication. It was also explained that after the operation he would be under close observation by the nursing staff, would be expected to deep-breathe and turn at intervals to prevent postoperative lung congestion, and would be kept free of pain with medication. He was told that he might be uncomfortable for a time, but that this was to be expected.

The next morning, the first of the preoperative medications was given by a student as ordered. At 11:30 A.M. the operating room clerk called the unit and the remaining medications were given. The patient complained of nausea thereafter and seemed very apprehensive, so the student stayed with him a while and encouraged him to take slow, deep breaths— an action that tends to have a relaxing effect if the breaths are deep and slow enough. He was also reassured that he would come back to the unit after operation and would be cared for by the nurses already familiar to him. He was assured that members of his family would be allowed to visit with him. Mr. T. dozed thereafter and seemed calm when he was taken from the unit to the operating room.

At operation, a left orchiectomy was done with excision of the spermatic cord to the inguinal ring. Blood loss was minimal (50 ml). The patient returned to the unit at 6 P.M., and a nurse made the following observations: color good, skin warm and dry, alert when aroused, vital signs stable, dressing dry and intact. After repositioning the patient, the postoperative orders were checked.

VS q 15 min till stable, then q 4 h x 4, then q shift
Clear fluids—advance to regular diet as tolerated
Bedrest tonight, OOB tomorrow, but *no* ambulation
Seconal 100 mg (po) h.s., PRN
Demerol 75–100 mg (IM) q 3–4 h, PRN for incisional pain
Hct in A.M.
MOM 45 ml (po) h.s., PRN

Turning, coughing, and deep breathing was done every hour during the evening and every 2 hours during the night. The patient was offered water or warm tea at these times—which he tolerated well in small amounts. His vital signs remained stable, but he had not voided; however, the nurse observed that he was comfortable and had no suprapubic distention. He spent an uneventful postoperative night except for complaints of incisional and back pain, for which he was promptly medicated. He voided 150 ml of dark amber urine at 3 A.M.

The morning of his first postoperative day, Mr. T. tolerated a full fluid breakfast well and was allowed to take his own bed bath—receiving assistance with a back wash and alcohol rub. Thereafter, he was medicated for pain and allowed to remain in bed for half an hour before being assisted out of bed into a chair. His dressing had remained dry and intact and his vital signs were stable.

The report of the pregnancy test was received; the results were negative. The patient continued to void dark amber urine, and his second postoperative day passed uneventfully. His diet was progressed to "regular." Mr. T. voiced no complaints of pain, and his emotional affect was good—he played cards with three of the other patients, watched television with a group of patients after requesting to be taken to the recreation room, and engaged in group conversation. He was also cheerful throughout the evening hours while his family visited him. No scrotal swelling was noted, his dressing remained intact, and he was voiding clear yellow urine. Vital-signs observations were discontinued, and his pain medication was renewed.

On the third postoperative day, the pathology report of the tissue specimen arrived on the unit; the tumor tissue was found to be moderately well demarcated. The tunica albuginea was intact; the spermatic cord had regular structure; and there was no evidence of tumor elements at the line of resection of the cord. A diagnosis of seminoma of the testicle had been confirmed and the length of resected spermatic cord was negative for evidence of malignancy.

The doctor reviewed the report and went in to

see the patient. He changed the dressing—noting that the wound was clean—and removed the primary skin sutures. Mr. T. was then told about the pathology findings—that he had had a tumor of the testicle, but was not told that it was malignant. The doctor emphasized the fact that preoperative x-rays had been good and this type of tumor tended to respond well when surgery and prophylactic radiotherapy were instituted. He advised Mr. T. that he would request a radiology consultation, that he would make the operative and x-ray findings known to the radiologist, and that recommendations would be made for a follow-up course of treatment.

The patient was visibly shaken after his discussion with the doctor. He refused his supper tray, and was observed "reading" during most of the early evening and "sleeping" through visiting hours. His parents spoke to the nurse just before leaving the unit; the doctor had told them that their son had a malignant tumor of the testicle and that, although no metastasis was visible on x-ray, microscopic metastasis might be present so that a course of radiotherapy would be instituted. He further told them that the prognosis was guarded as this is a serious disease in young adults, but that a five- to ten-year survival rate could be anticipated. Mr. T.'s parents wanted to know more about their son's tumor so, by way of reassurance, the nurse emphasized that seminomas are less prone to metastasize, are radiosensitive, and are not as malignant as other tumors of the testicle. It was also pointed out that removal before metastatic spread always holds a better prognosis than tumors discovered late in the course of their development, and that their son's negative chest and kidney films seemed to rule out metastatic spread. The nurse further stated that although it was true that there might be microscopic metastasis, they would do well to hope for the best. They seemed quite heartened thereafter.

The nurse then went to talk with the patient. His seclusive behavior had been observed and the nurse decided that an opportunity should be afforded to encourage him to verbalize his feelings and fears. She asked if he had spoken with the doctor during the time of the dressing change, Mr. T. responded that his major concern was whether the operation and x-ray treatment would "get it all out." The nurse reassured him that the doctor had removed all of the tumor and that his chest and kidney x-rays had been good. It was further explained that x-ray treatments were routine after this type of operation. He seemed relieved.

On the fourth postoperative day, ambulation orders were written, so the patient was allowed to walk about for short intervals during that day. He found the allowed increase in activity encouraging; he said he knew that he must be better. On the fifth postoperative day, he was permitted to ambulate as desired. He complained of backache at intervals, and even though this was not a severe or persistent discomfort the nurse recorded it on the chart and reported it to the doctor because such a complaint could be indicative of metastasis in a patient with testicular cancer. (This is especially true if the pain is on the affected side; the nurse should therefore attempt to ascertain where the "ache" is as well as how severe it is.)

The next day, with his chart, Mr. T. was taken by wheel chair to the Radiation Therapy Department. The radiologist started the course of treatment that day, and the patient returned to the unit with the following recommendation written on his chart:

A course of radiation to the abdominal lymph nodes is indicated, and his course of treatment in all will take about six weeks.

The patient experienced no illness after the treatment and was discharged two days later. He will have radiation therapy on an outpatient basis and during the course of treatment will be observed for evidence of untoward radiation sequelae such as bone-marrow depression and/or other blood dyscrasias. These patients seldom ask questions about the possibility of sterility, as they are young and rarely think to ask. The possibility of sterility secondary to radiation therapy is usually guarded against by carefully shielding the remaining testicle with a lead sheath during the treatments.

REFERENCES

1. Altman, B. L., and Malament, M. Carcinoma of the testis following orchiopexy. J. Urol., 97:498–504, 1967.
2. Campbell, M. F. Urology, 2nd ed., Philadelphia, W. B. Saunders Company, 1963, Vol. 2, pp. 1261–1283.
3. Collins, D. H., and Pugh, R. C. B. The pathology of testicular tumors. Brit. J. Urol., 36 (Suppl.): 1–111, 1964.
4. Creevy, C. D. Outline of Urology. New York, McGraw-Hill Book Company, 1964.
5. Dow, J. A., and Mostofi, F. K. Testicular tumors following orchiopexy. Southern Med. J., 60:193–195, 1967.
6. Hamm, F. C., and Weinberg, S. R. Urology in Medical Practice, 2nd ed. Philadelphia, J. B. Lippincott Co., 1962.
7. Kaufman, J. J. The diagnosis of testicular tumors. CA, 17:2–6, 1967.
8. ———Treatment of testicular tumors. CA, 17:54–59, 1967.
9. Patton, J. F., and Ross, G. The painful testicle. Hosp. Med. 3:24–40, 1967.
10. Richardson, J. F., and Leblanc, G. A. Treatment of testicular tumors: Analysis of 135 cases with 5-year follow-up. J. Urol. 93:717–720, 1965.
11. Robson, C. J. Testicular tumors: A collective review from the Canadian Academy of Urological Surgeons. J. Urol. 94:440–444, 1965.
12. Tavel, F. R., et al. Retroperitoneal lymph node dissection. J Urol., 89:241–245, 1963.
13. Wilson, T. H., et al. Aggressive approach to metastatic testicular teratocarcinoma. J. Urol., 96:239–242, 1966.

9

Two Diseases of the Kidney:
Tuberculosis and Cancer

THE PATIENT WITH TUBERCULOSIS
OF THE KIDNEY

Tuberculosis of the kidney is more common in men than in women, and patients presenting with the disease are usually between the ages of 20 and 40. Renal tuberculosis occurs secondary to pulmonary or gastrointestinal tuberculosis, even though the primary lesion may have been asymptomatic. Characteristically, an interval of time—anywhere from two to twenty years—passes between the formation of the primary lesion and the manifestation of renal disease. The primary focus is usually the lungs, and bacilli from such a focus enter the bloodstream during the initial infection; thus some degree of bilateral kidney involvement is usual. As the blood is filtered by the glomerular capillaries, the pathogens often invade the tubules. Thereafter, as caseation progresses, parenchymal tissue is destroyed and cavities become enlarged.

Bacilli and pus cells may appear in the urine anytime

after renal invasion, and the ureters and bladder can become infected subsequently. Ureteral strictures may result from such an infection, and bladder ulcerations accompanied by complaints of dysuria (in this instance experienced as burning on urination) and/or frequency may also occur. Painless, gross hematuria usually represents the erosion of minor blood vessels secondary to chronic tuberculous infection of the urinary tract, and pyuria of unknown origin (pyuria even when urine culture reveals an absence of pyogenic organisms) makes renal tuberculosis suspect. If the bacilli invade the prostatic ducts, prostate gland involvement ensues; it is the vas deferens, however, which transports the organisms to the epididymis.

The insidious onset of renal tuberculosis used to prevent early diagnosis of the disease. Few signs or symptoms appear before the occurrence of extensive tissue damage. Currently, however, the incidence of advanced cavity cases seen in institutions is diminishing. When pus cells are discovered in urine (pyuria) upon analysis—either during the course of a routine (or insurance) physical examination or during a hospital admission—the doctor is alerted to the possibility of genitourinary tuberculosis. A history of pulmonary or gastrointestinal tuberculosis and the development of urinary symptoms usually justifies a diagnostic work-up for renal tuberculosis. Further, the individual presenting with chronic, recurrent cystitis that does not respond satisfactorily to standard modalities of treatment is also a candidate for a tuberculosis work-up.

The diagnostic examination of the patient usually includes (1) a series of three 24-hour urine specimens for analysis for and concentration of *Mycobacterium tuberculosis*, (2) pyelography, and (3) cystoscopy (if the bladder has become infected). Culture *and* guinea-pig techniques are traditionally utilized for the examination of the urine. Some urologists are of the opinion that when culture and guinea-pig techniques are performed on a first-voided morning urine specimen, results comparable to the 24-hour urine determinations are obtained. However, more comparative clinical data regarding the results of both techniques will be needed before the traditional method is abandoned. Pyelograms may reveal calyces with ragged contours; these findings are indicative of tissue destruction secondary to tuberculosis. When cystoscopy is performed, in addition to the areas of inflammation that can be observed in the bladder mucosa, ulcers with surface exudate may be visible.

Great progress has been made in the treatment of renal tuberculosis. At one time, surgical excision of a kidney (nephrectomy) was the basic treatment of the disease. Today, combination drug therapy has provided an effective means of curing the disease—regardless of the amount of tissue damage or the presence of genitourinary complications—and surgical intervention is rarely indicated. Antituberculosis triple drug therapy is as effective against renal tuberculosis as it is for the treatment of tuberculosis elsewhere in the body. Izoniazid (INH), para-amino-salicylic acid (PAS), and streptomycin or Viomycin or Kanomycin have been used in combination as the long-term chemotherapeutic agents for the treatment of renal tuberculosis, the length of treatment having a direct relationship to the amount of tissue damage present. Currently, except when stubborn cases are encountered, the use of the injectable drugs is being replaced by oral medications such as ethionamide and cycloserine. Double drug therapy (INH 100 mg TID and PAS 5 g TID) extended over a two-year period is often instituted with good results; but, since PAS has unpleasant side-effects, patients sometimes omit it or take it irregularly. Triple drug therapy, therefore, yields better results because even if the PAS is not taken the patient will at least receive the benefit of two of the antimicrobial drugs specific for the treatment of tuberculosis. The student should recall that it is the free acid form of PAS that tends to cause gastrointestinal irritation and subsequent discomfort to the patient. Thus the sodium, calcium, or potassium salt of the drug is administered to patients; the sodium salt is most commonly used unless restricted sodium intake is indicated. Untoward reactions from triple drug therapy include dermatitis, fever, peripheral neu-

ritis, vertigo, and deafness. The student should therefore inquire about such symptoms whenever long-term triple drug
therapy is being implemented—*whether the patient has institu-
tional or outpatient status*. Pyridoxine is often given prophylac-
tically to prevent neuritis when INH is being administered for
extended periods of time; the student should remember that
when PAS is taken *after meals* the possibility of gastrointestinal
irritation is minimized. Although patients may become asymptomatic within a few weeks of the implementation of antituberculosis therapy, most urologists agree that treatment for
a minimum of two years is indicated to cure renal tuberculosis.

Isolation of the patient with active renal tuberculosis is
usually unnecessary unless other indications make sanatorium
care desirable. However, the patient should be placed on precautions and given simple, detailed instruction when self-care
is to be carried out at home. Clinical investigation has shown
that children who are exposed to the tuberculous urine of a par-
ent have a higher incidence of positive skin tests for tuberculosis than children in control groups. It is also known that
genital-tract tuberculosis can be transmitted through the semen.
Thus, to prevent the spread of genitourinary tuberculosis to
close contacts, precautions should be observed. The patient
should be told that when there has been contact with the
genitalia or with urine containing tuberculosis bacilli, thorough
handwashing should be done. Undergarments, linen, towels,
and washcloths used by the patient should be washed separately
from the rest of the family wash and—whenever possible—
allowed to dry in the sunlight and air. The patient should also
be cautioned to refrain from sexual intercourse while the tuberculosis bacilli are present in the urine because spread of the
disease to his sexual partner may occur.

Urologists agree that complete bedrest is unnecessary for
patients with renal tuberculosis. However, adequate rest should
be insured and excessive exertion avoided; the nurse can be of
invaluable help in assisting the patient with the planning of
his rest periods or daily activity schedule. Emotional support

is always indicated for the patient on prolonged limited activity and the nurse should explain the dynamics of the disease to him, encouraging him to verbalize fears and to ask for clarification when doubts arise. The doctor should be encouraged to discuss the range of activities the patient will be allowed to pursue so that irritability or dejection resulting from the boredom of inactivity may be prevented. Usually light activity requiring limited movement will be permitted during the active phase of the disease. The need for rest and adequate diet should also be stressed. A high protein diet should be encouraged. For the patient who lives alone or who is to be left alone during the day, meal planning may present a special problem. A conference with the dietician will prove beneficial and the nurse should endeavor to make this additional help available for the patient. When financial matters pose special problems for a patient, such difficulties may be mentioned during the course of conversations with the nurse, and consultation with a medical social worker may be indicated. Helpful information that would ordinarily not be available to the nurse or the patient may be obtained during such meetings, and few patients will perceive such interest adversely when the nurse acts as liaison. Interagency referral is an area of medical-service coordination that tends to be neglected by nursing personnel; however, such referral is inherent in the mandate given to today's nurse in the supervision of comprehensive patient care. This is particularly true for the patient with renal tuberculosis, and the nurse may be perceived as the expeditor of medical- and social-service referral.

If one of the injectable drugs is to be taken over an extended period of time, the patient or some member of his family should be taught to give the injection. Prior to discharge, enough time should be allotted for such instruction so that the patient (or family member) will have the opportunity to demonstrate his ability to give the injection and to ask questions about related concerns as they arise.

Although nephrectomy is now seldom needed because

antituberculosis drugs become concentrated in the nephrons, resulting in an almost 100 percent cure rate, segmental resection of the kidney (i.e., partial nephrectomy) may be indicated for the removal of a diseased but isolated portion of renal parenchyma. However, this is done infrequently even though complete eradication of the disease in such a portion can be effected in this manner. Of the three approaches utilized for renal operations—lumbar, transthoracic, and transabdominal—a *flank* or *lumbar* approach is preferred when partial nephrectomy is to be done for renal tuberculosis. This approach is utilized so that the peritoneal and pleural cavities will not be entered, thus eliminating the possibility of contamination to the structures contained there. Urinary infection is always brought under control prior to the procedure so that postoperative complications related to the spread of infection will be minimized. Triple drug therapy in the preoperative period tends to convert the target lesion into a form that will permit partial nephrectomy without the danger of contamination to surrounding tissue. Therefore the student should impress the patient with the importance of the medication and should remain present to offer encouragement while all of the pills are being taken whenever the reliability of the patient is doubtful. After partial nephrectomy is done, the postoperative care is similar to that elaborated in Chapter 5 concerning the patient with a flank incision. In addition, however, conscientious *observation for hemorrhage* must be stressed because the nature of the operation increases the possibility of postoperative bleeding; the parenchyma of a highly vascular structure must be incised to accomplish the removal of the tuberculous lesion.

When isolation and drainage of a scrotal lesion is done, or if a draining wound is present, contaminated dressings should be double-wrapped in paper bags before disposal. The soaking, thorough washing, and autoclaving of instruments subsequent to their use during dressing changes is sufficient for instrument care. After cystoscopy has been performed, the destruction of tuberculosis organisms by the cold sterilization method is most successfully effected by allowing the cystoscope to soak for 15 minutes (with all stop-cocks open) in a 10 percent formalin solution. Traditional cold sterilization methods are usually inadequate to kill mycobacterium tuberculosis. It should be remembered, however, that formalin is irritating to the skin and must be thoroughly washed from the instrument with a cleansing solution prior to being stored for future use.

Medical care during the period of prolonged triple drug therapy usually includes urinalysis at regular intervals, as well as IVP every six months, to enable the doctor to evaluate the status of the disease. (Films are often obtained as long as three years after all medication has been discontinued.) During the semiannual check-ups, cystoscopic examinations are not usually done. As previously mentioned, bladder contracture and/or ureteral stricture may occur following renal tuberculosis. The insertion of a ureteral catheter into both ureters may be done to accomplish either the dilatation of a ureteral stricture or the prevention of such stricture formation. However, it should be noted that catheters are not passed up ureters routinely.

The student making home visits should continually stress the principles of healthful living with these patients—especially the importance of diet, adequate rest, and *follow-up examinations*. Patients will frequently neglect the follow-up aspect when they are asymptomatic and when medications have been discontinued.

THE PATIENT WITH CANCER OF THE KIDNEY

Tumors of the kidney are usually malignant and may originate from any part of the structure: the capsule, cortex, medulla, or pelvis. Benign tumors may develop, but they are generally of little clinical significance and are usually discovered during the course of an autopsy. The only types of renal carcinomas that are of clinical significance are those which originate from embryonic tissue—appearing in infancy and childhood (Wilms' tumor); those which originate in the renal parenchyma of adults—occurring in the middle and late adult years (adenocarcinomas or hypernephromas); and epithelial tumors of the adult renal pelvis (papillary carcinomas). Of the three types mentioned, adenocarcinomas make up the largest percentage of renal tumors, and most of the growths requiring surgical intervention are of this type. Sarcomas of the kidney—both pure and mixed—are rare, but they possess a high degree of malignancy when they are present. This chapter will include a discussion of adenocarcinoma of the renal parenchyma and papillary carcinoma of the renal pelvis.

Most of the malignant tumors of the kidney grow insidiously and relatively fast. Many fail to cause symptoms and are discovered only accidentally during the course of a routine physical examination. Others develop into large tumors and cause the individual to manifest symptoms. The fact to be remembered, however, is that the signs and symtoms of renal carcinoma lack a distinguishable pattern; thus the prognosis is usually poor unless some early indication leads a doctor to conduct a thorough diagnostic work-up for renal neoplasm.

When in the clinical situation or when reviewing the literature, the student will notice that adenocarcinoma of the kidney is also referred to as renal cell carcinoma, hypernephroma, Grawitz's tumor, and clear cell carcinoma. The student need only remember that all these terms refer to the malignant neoplasm of the adult kidney.

Characteristics, Signs, Symptoms of Adenocarcinoma of the Renal Parenchyma

Adenocarcinoma of the kidney is usually found in individuals over the age of 50. It is generally believed that these neoplasms originate from mature renal parenchymal tissue, even though histologic findings have led some urologists to speculate that they may arise from benign renal adenomas. Because this disease occurs more often in men (with almost twice the frequency of its occurrence in women), other urologists suspect a hormonal relationship. These tumor masses are usually found occupying an area near the upper or lower pole of either kidney; however, it should be noted that tumor masses have also been found at the center of the parenchyma. Tumor growth causes the compression of surrounding renal tissue as well as the displacement and distortion of calyces and the renal pelvis. Blood vessel displacement as well as invasion of the renal vein often occurs, and metastasis to the liver, lungs, and long bones by way of the bloodstream are characteristic. Since metastasis often occurs early in the course of the disease and bears little relationship to the size of the tumor, symptomatology from distant structures (especially the lungs) may herald the presence of the disease. Bony metastasis occurs chiefly in the vertebrae, pelvis, femur, and humerus. Extension of the tumor to the lumbar lymph nodes surrounding the renal pedicle may also occur, and this lymphatic network may serve to extend the tumor to the paraaortic lymph nodes.

It cannot be said that there are signs which specifically indicate the presence of an adenocarcinoma or that the adenocarcinoma initiates a characteristic set of symptoms. At one time it was thought that the triad of (1) gross, intermittent hematuria; (2) dull, dragging back pain; and (3) a palpable or visible mass in the flank was diagnostic of adenocarcinoma of the kidney. However, it is generally agreed today that this classic triad is seldom encountered as part of the presenting symptom complex. Painless, intermittent hematuria is the most common presenting symptom even though bleeding may be microscopic or gross, continuous or periodic. Hematuria usually occurs late in the course of the disease, and the interval between bleeding episodes may extend for weeks or even months. The period at which bleeding occurs tends to bear a direct relationship to the location of the tumor. Bleeding will be seen to occur early when tumors originate in the kidney pelvis, but will not be manifested with adenocarcinomas of the renal parenchyma until penetration of the pelvis or extension into the general collecting system occurs. Hematuria may also be indicative of invasion of the intrarenal circulation. Large clots in the bladder may cause obstruction at the bladder neck and result in a presenting symptom of urinary retention. In these cases, the bladder becomes suspect as the source of the hematuria.

In about half of the presenting patients, pain is experienced and reported as being either sharp and/or excruciating or dull and nondescript. The passage of clots or tumor tissue down the ureter will cause the patient to experience pain which is similar to renal colic, whereas dull, dragging pain felt in the flank or in the back is usually related to the weight of the tumor, the perirenal extension of the tumor, the compression of the ureter, hemorrhaging into the tumor, or irritation to the nerve root. Distention of the renal capsule will also cause the patient to experience considerable pain. Regarding the palpation of a mass, many tumors develop in an area which prohibits the palpation of a nodule or other irregularity—for example, the posterior surface or the upper pole of the kidney. Although many patients present with a mass which can be felt, this is a relatively late symptom. Palpation of an abdominal mass is rare, but patients have been known to seek medical advice after self-palpation of a renal mass.

Nonurologic symptoms are frequently experienced by patients with adenocarcinoma of the kidney. These include gastrointestinal complaints, unexplained low-grade fever, vascular complications, and the symptoms associated with metastasis. Varying degrees of anemia secondary to blood loss, the metastatic process, and/or anorexia may also develop. Gastrointestinal complaints secondary to renal malignancy often resemble symptoms of peptic ulcers or gall-bladder disease and may include varying degrees of nausea and vomiting, abdominal discomfort, and anorexia. It is believed that reflex action or displacement (or invasion) of adjacent organs is responsible for these symptoms. The patient may also present with a history of continuous weight loss, increased weakness, general malaise, and lethargy. On the other hand, unexplained low-grade fever may be the only presenting symptom of renal malignancy, and it is found to occur with significant frequency. Hemorrhaging within the tumor mass with subsequent absorption of hematin, toxins from the tumor itself, or infection associated with the tumor may account for the fever. Occasionally, metastasis to the brain occurs and, when these metastatic lesions involve the body's heat-regulating center, fever may result. Other symptoms associated with metastasis include a painful or swollen femur, a pathologic fracture of a long bone, or a cough or dyspnea caused by a chest lesion. Obstruction of the vena cava may result in vascular complications such as leg edema and/or dilatation of the abdominal veins. These are serious complications and serve as an index of inoperability.

Papillary Carcinoma of the Renal Pelvis

In contrast to adenocarcinoma of the renal parenchyma, papillary carcinoma of the renal pelvis accounts for only a small percentage (less than 10 percent) of all renal malignancies. This disease originates in the mucosa of the renal pelvis and/or calyces, and it looks like a colony of nipplelike protuberances—resembling tumors found in the bladder. Frequently patients with these lesions have a history of bladder cancer. Metastases to distant organs are not characteristic of these tumors, although the regional lymph nodes and the renal vein may be involved.

Gross, painless hematuria is frequently the earliest symptom manifested. When pain is present it usually simulates the extreme discomfort of renal colic and is initiated when blood clots or tumor particles travel down the ureters. If the lesion originates near the ureteropelvic junction, hydronephrosis, hydrocalyx, or even nonfunctioning of the kidney may develop and the patient will usually complain of a dull, aching pain in the flank.

Diagnosis and Treatment of Renal Malignancies

Several procedures may be utilized to confirm a diagnosis of renal carcinoma. X-ray techniques include a flat plate of the abdomen, an excretory urogram (for example, the IVP—an x-ray taken while the kidneys are excreting dye and urine, hence the name *excretory urogram*), nephrotomography, and renal angiography. A flat plate of the abdomen often reveals kidney enlargement and/or any significant bulge of its contour. The position of the kidney is also important; a lowered position is of special significance because the size of the tumor mass may cause downward displacement. This general, gross inspection is limited, however, and more conclusive evidence may be obtained from an excretory urogram or from a retrograde pyelogram. (Since the kidneys are not required to excrete the dye deposited in the renal pelvis during the retrograde procedure, *the retrograde pyelogram is not considered to be an excretory urogram.*)

The IVP will accurately reveal a space-occupying lesion within the renal parenchyma because—as the dye is filtered through the action of parenchymal structures—the substance of the kidney is opacified. In addition, filling defects (the term used when dye cannot be visualized within a structure or cavity) and any changes in the configuration of the calyces and/or kidney pelvis will be demonstrated. Many urologists agree that cystoscopy should be performed during a bleeding episode so that the exact source may be ascertained; and, although retrograde pyelograms are not essential to the diagnosis of carcinoma of the renal parenchyma, in these instances retrograde studies are usually done. These studies are particularly helpful in demonstrating the signs characteristic of the presence of a tumor mass—for example, the lobulated outline and increased size of the kidney, the change in the normal contour of the affected calyces or pelvis, and any filling defect in the calyces. It should be mentioned that in almost all instances the evidence from either IVP or the retrograde pyelogram will be sufficient to establish a diagnosis of carcinoma of the renal pelvis. Instead of a filling defect within the substance of the renal parenchyma being of significance, however, it is the presence of a filling defect within the collecting system (the kidney pelvis or calyces) that is significant. The various degrees of hydronephrosis and/ or hydrocalyx revealed will also help to establish the diagnosis. As tuberculosis tends to mimic cancer of the renal pelvis, 24-hour urine specimens for bacteriologic study for the presence of the tuberculosis bacillus are usually obtained to rule out that possibility. Urine cytology may be done also.

Renal arteriography outlines the renal circulation and will demonstrate renal neoplasms. It is accomplished with a radiopaque dye which is injected intrarterially into large vessels situated near the renal vessels. Two techniques may be utilized: either (1) the retrograde femoral technique in which contrast media is injected into the femoral artery to define the arterial blood supply to the tumor or (2) the lumbar needle puncture technique in which the contrast media (radiopaque dye) is introduced directly into the aorta above the renal arteries. Renal arteriography is particularly useful in assisting the urologist to rule out the possibility of the mass's being a benign renal cyst. Malignant tumors characteristically have a rich vascular supply, while benign cystic tumors do not. Thus vascularized tissue within the renal parenchyma will be opacified and a pooling of the contrast media in the area of the tumor mass may be visualized if a malignancy is present (see Fig. 1). On the other hand, if a benign cystic tumor is present, the cyst will fail to opacify and arteries will be seen to surround the mass (see Fig. 2). This occurs because cystic masses tend to produce a stretching and distortion of the arterial vessels around them. It should be noted, however, that the walls of a small but significant percentage of renal cysts have been found to contain cancer cells. Therefore, most urologists

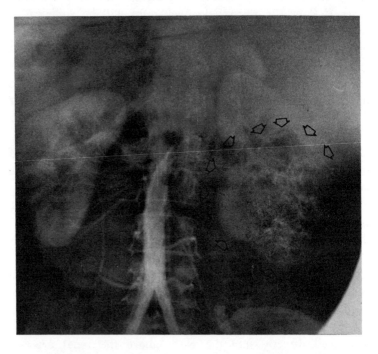

Fig. 1. Hypernephroma of the kidney (clear cell carcinoma or Grawitz's tumor). This femoral arteriogram demonstrates the pooling of the contrast media in the area of the tumor mass (note the arrow). Malignant tumors characteristically have a rich vascular supply. Note the regular contour of the unaffected kidney. (Courtesy of Department of Radiodiagnosis, St. Vincent's Hospital and Medical Center of New York.)

will assume that a renal cyst is malignant until they obtain evidence that it is benign. The preparation of the patient is the same as the preparation for an IVP. If a femoral approach has been utilized, the student should be careful to *lift up the dressing* when checking the puncture site after the patient's return to the unit. Hematoma formation may occur even when there is no blood on the dressing. When a discolored "lump" does seem to be forming under the surface of the skin, pressure exerted over the puncture site (accomplished by pressing two or three fingers of one hand on the dressing for a few minutes) will stop the oozing of blood from the artery in most cases. However, if—during the course of subsequent observation—the hardened area seems to enlarge, the doctor should be notified. The patient should also be encouraged to force fluids to make up for the period of dehydration prior to the procedure.

Although special radiographic procedures are seldom necessary to establish a diagnosis of carcinoma of the renal pelvis, other diagnostic x-ray procedures may be needed to establish or confirm a diagnosis of carcinoma within the renal parenchyma. Nephrotomography is such a procedure. It has been valuable in revealing small tumors which might otherwise go unnoticed. Serial films of different sections of the renal parenchyma are taken during this procedure. Thus the urologist is able to view different levels of renal tissue. The preparation of the patient is the same as that for IVP. A newer technique of renal photoscanning is also being used currently by some urologists for the detection of space-occupying lesions of the renal parenchyma. It is accomplished through the intravenous injection of radioactive mercury. Subsequent to the injection, the renal parenchyma is scanned for radioactivity because usually there is good, uniform concentration of this radioisotope in a normal kidney. When a space-occupying lesion is present in the renal parenchyma, however, concentration of the radioisotope is negligible and the renal mass is usually outlined. This procedure is considered to be particularly valuable when bilateral parenchy-

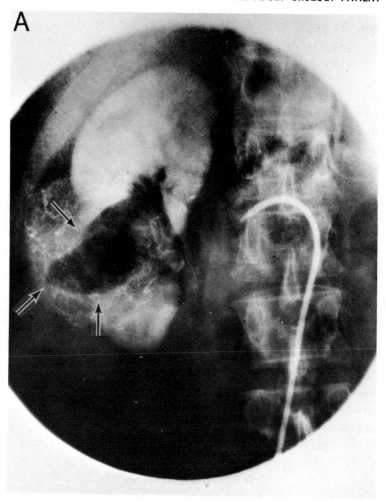

Fig. 2A. A benign cystic tumor of the Kidney. A. Note how the arteries **surround** the mass. A cystic tumor has no vascular supply.

mal lesions are suspected. A skeletal or metastatic series is usually obtained to determine the presence of metastatic lesions once the diagnosis has been made. This will seem logical if the student will recall that radical treatment is seldom used when

B

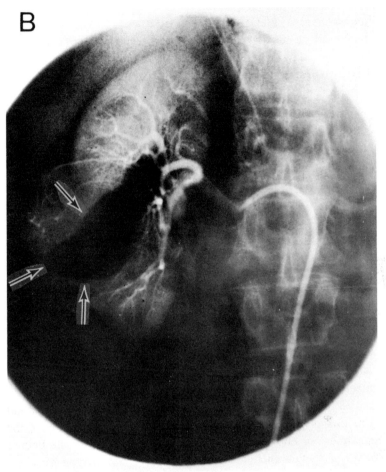

Fig. 2B. A cystic tumor does, however, produce stretching of the arterial vessel around it. (A and B Courtesy of Department of Radiodiagnosis, St. Vincent's Hospital and Medical Center of New York.)

metastatic lesions have developed. The series usually includes x-ray examination of the chest, skull, spine, and long bones.

A urinalysis obtained during the course of the diagnostic work-up will usually reveal hematuria. Investigators also discovered that there was an elevation in the urinary lactic dehydrogenase (LDH) concentration of almost all patients diagnosed as having renal or bladder cancer. However, LDH levels are now thought to be useless. Since the elevation in LDH concentration occurs *prior to* the manifestation of symtoms specifically related to the tumor, it is believed that this test may prove invaluable for the early detection of renal and bladder malignancies.

A renal-function test (usually the PSP test described in Chapter 6) generally completes the diagnostic work-up of the patient. This is done in addition to the IVP to ascertain the function of the unaffected kidney. It seems appropriate at this juncture to stress the nurse's responsibility for the success of this test. The collection bottles for the urine specimens should be clearly labeled with the patient's name *and* the time that the specimen is to be obtained within the 2-hour interval of the test. The nurse should also be sure to explain to the patient that he should make every effort to urinate at the intervals specified so that the test will not have to be repeated.

Treatment usually depends on the results of the various diagnostic procedures. The size and mobility of the kidney is another important factor in determining the type of treatment that will be used; the general condition and age of the patient are also considered. If there is no metastasis and renal function is good in the unaffected kidney, nephrectomy is the treatment of choice. If the lesion is confined within the boundaries of the parenchyma and—during exploratory surgical exposure—the exterior surface of the kidney appears normal, nephrectomy is again the treatment of choice. When severe hemorrhage cannot be stopped, nephrectomy may be the only course of treatment open to the urologist—despite the presence of metastases. Nephrectomy is often done in the presence of metastases because spontaneous regression of the latter has been described in cases where the primary tumor was excised. In some instances, nephrectomy may also be performed to effect the relief of pain. As previously stated, *radical treatment* is rarely done when metastatic lesions are present. Such radical treatment would include nephrectomy and extensive node dissection. Many urologists believe that extension of the tumor into the renal vein should not be a deterrent to nephrectomy and the removal of the growth from the vessel. Nephrectomy is usually done—even in the presence of lung metastasis—whenever the mass is removable; however, if the tumor is fixed to other structures such as the liver, spleen, aorta, or diaphragm, removal is usually not attempted. Generally, it may be said that nephrectomy (with or without removal of the ureter) is the preferred treatment for adenocarcinoma of the renal parenchyma; nephroureterectomy (with excision of the periureteral portion of the bladder) is the preferred treatment for papillary carcinoma of the renal pelvis because this tumor spreads along the ureter to the UV (ureterovesical) junction.

Since most malignancies of the adult kidney are radioresistant, radiation therapy is not part of the routine postoperative treatment. It may be employed, however, to effect the temporary regression of the primary growth in inoperable cases. Some urologists believe that this accomplishes a temporary diminution in the size of the mass as well as a reduction in its vascularity. It should be noted, however, that this point of view is controversial.

During the postoperative period, the student should make a conscientious effort to discover what the patient has been told about body functioning after the loss of one kidney, and the student should endeavor to reinforce and add to this knowledge. Fears and anxieties regarding the consequences of the removal of one kidney tend to build in the patient as the day of operation approaches. Most patients know that the kidneys are essential to life, but they usually do not understand how one kidney is able to do the work of two. It should be explained, therefore, that in each adult kidney there is much more tissue available for the excretion of waste products than is actually required to perform that function. This should help the patient to appreciate that the loss of one kidney will not represent a threat to his life or in any way reduce his living status to a level of semiinvalidism. Further, the positive aspects of the situation should be stressed by reassuring the patient—when renal function in the unaffected kidney is adequate—that tests of the performance of the remaining kidney were good, indicating that it will be able to meet the demands of his body during the course of his life.

Surgical Management of Malignancies of the Kidney

Three operative approaches are commonly utilized to accomplish the surgical removal of the kidney when carcinoma has been diagnosed: the transabdominal (or transperitoneal) approach, the transthoracic (or thoracoabdominal) approach, and the lumbar (or flank) approach. Whenever nephrectomy is being performed for renal malignancy—regardless of the approach employed—the kidney is widely resected in order to remove all of the tissue that may be involved. Early isolation and occlusion of either the renal vein or the entire renal pedicle is done before the renal mass is manipulated so that the intravenous infusion of tumor cells will be prevented. If exploration reveals involvement of the renal vein or abdominal vena cava, extensive surgical procedures are seldom performed.

The transperitoneal approach will not be discussed in detail here because it is most frequently used for the excision of renal tumors in children. However, it should be mentioned that when this approach is utilized in adults, there exists a possibility of the pleura being perforated. Therefore, the student should be alert to the symptoms of pneumothorax: sudden, sharp chest pains; dyspnea; anxiety; and accelerated pulse rate. When pneumothorax occurs, a high Fowler's position should be maintained for the patient and—after the doctor has been notified—oxygen and a thoracotomy set should be mobilized for emergency use. The patient will appear very frightened during this experience, so the student should make every effort to remain calm. The patient should not be left alone, and the student should remember that the responsibility of "presence" and of offering words of reassurance and comfort are equally as important as assisting the doctor during the emergency procedures. The student will find that—except in the most extraordinary situations—help from staff members is usually abundant at these times. The transthoracic approach is usually preferred for the excision of large renal tumors in adults. By converting the pleural and abdominal cavities into one operative field, unexcelled exposure of even the superior pole of the kidney is afforded. Ribs are resected, the thoracic cavity is entered, and the diaphragm is incised along its fibers. An extension of the midline abdominal incision permits retraction of the abdominal viscera covering the great vessels; this facilitates extensive visualization of the renal pedicle and of the lymph nodes around the aorta and vena cava. This approach also facilitates the resection of the retroperitoneal fascia and metastatic lymph nodes following the removal of the kidney. At the completion of the procedure, the chest and abdominal cavity are closed in layers and thoracotomy tubes are left to drain the pleural cavity. These tubes are subsequently attached to underwater drainage apparatus to prevent pneumothorax, but they are removed as soon as the lungs demonstrate full expansion. It should be noted that some surgeons do not use thoracotomy tubes.

There are two aspects of the transthoracic approach that warrant special discussion: (1) the fact that one or two ribs may be resected to accomplish the procedure and that (2), postoperatively, the patient may return to the unit with a chest tube in place. Because of the resected rib (or ribs), coughing will be difficult for such a patient and much encouragement and *mechanical support* will be necessary if he is to be expected to accomplish the tasks of deep breathing and coughing. After a draw sheet or large towel has been positioned about the chest to splint the operative area, the patient should be told to press the upper part of the arm on the affected side toward the body while bringing the forearm across the waist—the hand resting at the side. The student should then grasp the mechanical support firmly at the back and encourage the patient to take several slow, deep breaths and then to cough. This should be done *hourly* during the waking hours of the first postoperative day and every 2 hours during the night. Thereafter, although the patient should be encouraged to deep-breathe and cough frequently without assistance, the student should assist the patient in the manner described on a 2-hour basis until the lungs are fully expanded and the chest is clear. This serves as a supervisory measure to insure that the patient is doing the ventilation exercises correctly and effectively. The approximate amount, color, and character of the sputum should also be recorded. Regarding the presence of the chest tube, two clamps should be placed conspicuously at the bedside—either clipped to the linen at the head of the bed or held in place on the bedside table by a single strip of adhesive tape. The care of the chest tubes and precautions to be observed when caring for a patient with underwater chest drainage is pertinent to this situation as well. However, it should be remembered that before any part of the drainage apparatus is disconnected (for whatever reason), *the nurse should double-clamp the chest catheter close to the patient's body*. If the chest tube should be pulled out accidentally, the first course of action should be to *cover up the opening* and then notify the doctor.

The lumbar or flank approach has already been discussed in Chapter 5. It should be mentioned, however, that this approach accomplishes the removal of the affected kidney without necessitating involvement of the peritoneal and pleural cavities; *it is most commonly used when active infection is present*, so that the possibility of contamination of those cavities is eliminated.

Two observations crucial to the progress of the patient following renal operations for malignancy are observation of the vital signs and observation of the urinary output. The possibility of internal hemorrhaging into the retroperitoneal space is present because the wide resection of the kidney usually leaves only a ligated stub of the normally short renal vessels remaining. Often, an increase in pulse rate and/or restlessness even after medication has been given could be the earliest indications of internal bleeding. When these signs are accompanied by a gradual drop in blood pressure, the doctor should be notified. The student should always check to be certain that the patient has blood on call for emergency use during the early postoperative period, and a dressing set together with a knife and long-handled hemostat should be available for emergency use. If hemorrhage occurs, a blood transfusion is usually started and the patient is returned to the operating room. Observation of the dressing, conscientious recording of the amount and character of the drainage present, and reinforcement when necessary should be carried out in the same manner that has been taught for other types of surgical procedures.

As for the recording of urinary output, many patients are returned from surgery with indwelling transurethral catheters, so that an accurate record of output may be kept. The *color and amount* of urine should be recorded; often hourly measurement is requested (especially when output is found to be highly concentrated and limited). If an indwelling catheter has not been inserted and the patient has not voided within an interval of 8 to 10 hours following operation, the doctor should be notified so that the patient may be catheterized. In some instances, the patient may be uncomfortable and unable to void prior to the designated maximum time allowed. When this occurs, the doctor should be notified so that immediate catheterization may be performed for the relief of discomfort.

Regardless of the approach utilized, positioning of the patient in the early postoperative period is important: he must be turned frequently. There are two schools of thought about the positioning of a patient after nephrectomy. Some urologists request that the patient be positioned toward the unaffected side so that reexpansion of the lung on the affected side will be facilitated. Others will specify that the patient be positioned on the affected side so that the space previously occupied by the kidney will be obliterated. Both theories are geared toward minimizing the possibility of postoperative complications, and the student should check the orders to learn the doctor's preference. If specific positioning instructions are absent, it should be assumed that the patient may be turned from side to side.

As a precautionary measure against reflex paralytic ileus, the patient may return to the unit with a nasogastric tube to suction. The added distress of abdominal distention, nausea, and vomiting may be avoided through this action. The tube is usually kept in place for only a short period of time and the student would do well to remember that oral fluids should be offered in limited amounts until bowel sounds are audible (without the use of a stethoscope) or the patient begins to pass gas per rectum. When gastric suction is not used during the early postoperative period, oral fluids must be given cautiously because the activity of the gastrointestinal tract is usually sluggish at this time.

Throughout the postoperative period, words of encouragement about the progress of the patient's status and reassurance that the discomforts being experienced are transitory give comfort to most patients. *Simple explanations* about the reasons for the various treatments will tend to make the patient more cooperative, and brief reports of progress to one close family member will often provide the support needed to enable the family to help in efforts to allay the patient's apprehensions. At the end of the course of hospitalization, the patient should be given some guidelines regarding self-care when he goes home. To this end, the importance of maintaining an adequate fluid intake should be stressed and the patient should be cautioned to limit his alcoholic intake because of the diuretic effect of

lcoholic beverages. The patient should be encouraged to pur-
ue suggested measures for the treatment of any respiratory in-
ection promptly because, if neglected, even a cold might
esult in prolonged immobilization and its associated hazards to
he urinary tract. In addition, the patient should be warned
against doing heavy lifting or straining for a 2-month period
ollowing discharge. The need for follow-up periodic cystoscopic examinations should be stressed for the patient who has
been treated for papillary carcinoma of the renal pelvis; such
examinations facilitate the early detection of subsequent papil-
omas of the bladder.

Other Treatment Modalities

For those lesions which are radiosensitive, radiation over
metastatic sites is employed. Radiation over the resected area
is also employed postoperatively for those malignancies which
are found to be radiosensitive. The results of chemotherapy
have not been encouraging for the most part. Nitrogen mustard
has had little effect, and halogenated pyrimidine (5-FU) is of
limited value. However, research continues for drugs that will
prove less toxic to the body in general and more effective at
the target site.

REFERENCES

1. Ansell, J. S. Nephrectomy and nephrostomy. Amer. J. Nurs.,
   58:1394–1396, 1958.
2. Antonio, D. Management of renal tumors. Philipp. J. Surg.,
   19:321–325, 1964.
3. Becker, J. A., et al. Renal tuberculosis: Role of nephrotomography and angiography. J. Urol., 100:415–419, 1968.
4. Besley, J. K. Malignancies in the kidneys. Med. Serv. J.
   Canada, 20:978–804, 1964.

5. Borromeo, V. H. J. Symptoms and diagnosis of renal tumor. Philipp. J. Surg., 19:318–320, 1964.
6. Carr, D. T. The treatment of renal tuberculosis. Med. Clin N. Amer., 50:1137–1139, 1966.
7. Committee on Therapy, American Thoracic Society, Medical Section of the National Tuberculosis Association: The present status of genitourinary tuberculosis. Amer. Rev. Resp. Dis., 92:505–507, 1965.
8. Cox, C. E., and Smith, D. R. Neoplasms of the kidney and adrenal gland. Calif. Med., 100:351–357, 1964.
9. Ewert, E. E., et al. Hypernephroma: The great imitator. Med. Clin. N. Amer., 47:431–436, 1963.
10. Foster, R. S. Selective renal angiography in clinical urology. J. Urol., 90:631–641, 1963.
11. Gow, J. G. Renal calcification in genito-urinary tuberculosis. Brit. J. Surg., 52:283–288, 1965.
12. Gray, C. P., and Biorn, C. L. Partial nephrectomy—indications and technique. Arch. Surg., 94:798–802, 1967.
13. Greene, L. F., et al. Nephrotomography in urologic diagnosis. J. Urol., 91:184–189, 1964.
14. Khoury, E. N. Thoraco--abdominal approach in lesions of the kidney, adrenal and testis. J. Urol., 96:631–634, 1966.
15. Kiely, J. M. Hypernephroma—the internist's tumor. Med. Clin. N. Amer., 50:1067–1083, 1966.
16. Lattimer, J. K. Modern treatment of renal tuberculosis. Sem. Rep., 4:2–9, 1959.
17. ——— Renal tuberculosis. New Eng. J. Med., 273:208–211, 1965.
18. National Tuberculosis and Respiratory Disease Association: Diagnostic Standards and Classification of Tuberculosis. New York Tuberculosis and Health Association, 1969.
19. Taufic, M. R. Nursing the patient after nephrectomy. Amer. J. Nurs., 58:1397–1398, 1958.

10

The Patient with a Bladder Tumor

Tumors of the bladder occur three times more frequently in men than in women, and the incidence seems to increase with age. They are most commonly found in individuals over the age of 50, and rank second to prostatic tumors in frequency (the latter being the most common of all genitourinary neoplasms).

The etiology of the pathogenesis is obscure. A causal relationship has been proved between exposure to beta-naphthylamine and the development of bladder tumors. It was noted that workers in the aniline dye industry who had either ingested beta-naphthylamine or inhaled its fumes subsequently developed bladder cancer. However, it must be noted that the number of patients presenting with a history of this kind of contact comprise only a small sample of the total population of new cases of patients with bladder cancer. Ingestion, inhalation, or cutaneous applications of other chemical compounds are also believed to cause bladder tumors. It is thought that these compounds may gain entrance into the body through certain foodstuffs, medicines, cosmetics, and clothing. Chronic inflammation from irritation or recurrent infection has also been suggested as a possible cause of bladder cancer. Speculation has been that the chronic inflammatory process could stimulate the transitional epithelium to produce certain intermediate changes necessary for the development of a bladder tumor. Further, since it is known that the carcinogen is transported by the urine, residual urine containing such a substance provides increased probability of tumor inducement.

THE URINARY BLADDER

The bladder wall has four layers. Progressing from the outermost layer inward, the *outer layer is partly advenitia* and *partly serosa*. It is a reflection of the peritoneum and covers the upper part of the lateral surfaces of the bladder as well as the superior surface. The *muscular layer*—immediately adjacent to the serous layer—is made up of three strata: the inner longitudinal, middle circular, and outer longitudinal. At the bladder neck, the circular fibers converge to form a thick layer or sphincter muscle. This sphincter muscle is called the *internal urinary sphincter*. In the normal state, the internal sphincter is contracted. It relaxes when enough urine has accumulated to warrant emptying of the bladder. The *submucosa* is the next layer of the bladder wall. It is composed of connective tissue and joins the innermost layer of the bladder wall—the *mucous membrane*—and the muscular layer. The *inner mucous membrane*, which lines the bladder, is composed of transitional epithelium. It is continuous with the mucosal layer of the lumen of the ureters and urethra. The connection of the mucous membrane to the underlying muscular layer is loose throughout most of the internal bladder surface and assumes the appearance of a series of folds or wrinkles when the bladder is empty. There is a small triangular area at the bladder neck, however, that is always smooth. In this area the mucous membrane is firmly attached to the underlying muscular layer. This smooth area is known as the *trigone* of the bladder. The two ureters enter the bladder wall in a downward oblique angle and their slitlike orifices within the bladder mark the outer boundaries of the base of the trigone. The urethral orifice at the bladder neck marks the apex of the trigone.

Pathologic Characteristics of Tumors

The majority of bladder tumors arise in the mucous membrane layer of the bladder wall. Therefore, the cells comprising these tumors have characteristics similar to transitional cell epithelium. They are papillary in nature. Nonepithelial tumors represent only a small percentage of bladder tumors. For the purposes of this text, all of the mucosal and submucosal tumors are considered to be superficial and early infiltrating growths, respectively. Tumors which invade muscle and penetrate through muscle to paravesical fat are considered infiltrating. The depth of the bladder wall penetration is generally the criterion which urologists utilize when evaluating the course of treatment to be followed. It should be noted that tumors which involve a large segment of the bladder wall may be papillary or infiltrating in nature.

In most instances, tumors of the urinary bladder originate near the bladder floor. The ureteral and urethral orifices are often obstructed, and stasis of urine tends to increase the incidence of complications both during and after treatment. The tumors usually begin as abnormal cellular proliferations of the mucous membrane lining. Benign tumors protrude from the mucosal surface as small nipplelike (papillomatous) outgrowths. The submucosal layer provides these cells with blood vessels and the connective tissue of that layer often extends into the growths. These noninfiltrating benign tumors occur as single or multiple outgrowths which tend to recur at new sites in the bladder after local destruction has been accomplished. It is believed that epithelial cells from the tumor's growth are readily implanted in the operative field, producing local recurrences of the tumor. It has also been noted that these benign tumors may undergo malignant degeneration with successive recurrences. Nonepithelial infiltrating tumors seldom invade the bladder wall beyond the muscular layer. Transitional cell and squamous cell tumors fall into this group. They occur less frequently than the papillary growths and are malignant. The squamous cell carcinoma is considered highly malignant.

Adenocarcinomas and sarcomas are rare. When they occur, however, they tend to infiltrate deeply into the bladder wall and beyond. Although a palpable suprapubic mass is rarely noted, its occurrence is sometimes associated with these tumors. Bladder neck and either unilateral or bilateral ureteral obstruction may also occur. With extension outside of the bladder, the tumors may adhere to the pelvic wall, the pelvic organs, or to the abdominal wall—resulting in extravesical obstruction.

The Diagnosis of Tumor

Although the earliest indication of a bladder tumor is a transient episode of hematuria, gross painless hematuria is the presenting symptom in approximately 80 percent of the patients. The diagnosis of a bladder tumor may be established during a cystoscopic examination performed because of an episode of hematuria. However, gross painless hematuria may be either a presenting symptom or it may occur secondary to stimulation of a quiescent bladder tumor during pelvic examination, or during a digital rectal examination or abdominal palpation, or following proctoscopy. Therefore, when postexamination hematuria occurs, the nurse should always notify the doctor immediately. Bleeding resulting from the presence of a bladder tumor is not always visible upon gross inspection of the urine. It should be noted that microscopic hematuria detected during a routine urinalysis is also of significance.

In addition to hematuria, bladder irritability simulating an infectious process in the bladder may also occur because the tumor is a foreign body. If an infectious process has developed secondary to the tumor development, the patient may complain of frequency, urgency, pain, pyuria, or burning on urination. Obstruction at the vesical outlet may result either in the kind of complaints characteristic of early prostatism or the complications characteristic of advanced prostatism: hydroureter, hydronephrosis, and/or pyelonephritis. The patient may even present with azotemic or uremic symptoms which are secondary to impaired renal function. Complaints of pain in the bladder, rectum, pelvis, flank, back, or legs usually indicate an advanced disease process. Fever and severe flank pain usually indicate renal infection. Complaints of weakness and weight loss may result from either severe infection or the consequences of metastasis. Venous obstruction is manifested by leg edema. On the other hand, bladder tumors often fail to cause symptoms because of their location. By the time tumor growth and tissue invasion have developed sufficiently to cause symptoms, a great deal of time may have elapsed.

Fortunately, an early diagnosis of an asymptomatic bladder tumor may be made as the result of evaluation of an excretory urogram or through visualization during a cystoscopic examination being performed for other reasons. During evaluation of an IVP, a filling defect noted in the bladder often alerts the doctor to the possibility of the presence of a bladder tumor. However, direct visualization (through endoscopy or cystoscopy) and biopsy are necessary to confirm the diagnosis. Once the tumor has been visualized cystoscopically, an adequate biopsy must be obtained to confirm the diagnosis (see Fig. 1). The pathology report aids the doctor in deciding upon the proper therapeutic course. The muscular layer of the bladder is usually included with the tumor specimen during biopsy. This permits

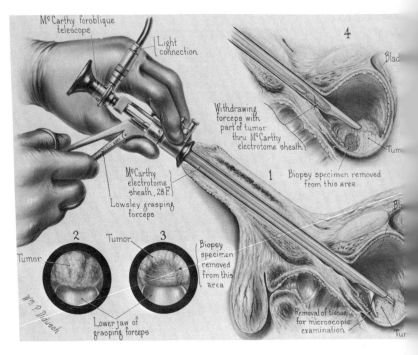

Fig. 1. Biopsy of a bladder tumor. (Courtesy of the American Cystoscope Makers, Inc., Pelham Manor, New York.)

an approximation of the degree of bladder wall infiltration. The degree of tumor invasion may also be estimated through the *bimanual pelvic examination* (see Fig. 2). In the male patient, this involves abdominorectal palpation; in the female patient it involves abdominovaginal palpation. Such an examination is usually done after the patient is anesthetized prior to cystoscopic examination. It is of great importance in assessing the size as well as the extent of the tumor growth.

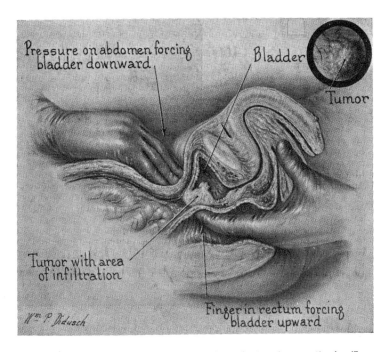

Pressure on abdomen forcing bladder downward

Bladder

Tumor

Tumor with area of infiltration

Wm. P. Didusch

Finger in rectum forcing bladder upward

Fig. 2. Bimanual palpation of bladder in male patient under anesthesia. (From Jewett. *In* Campbell, ed. Urology, 2nd ed. 1963. Courtesy of W. B. Saunders Co.)

Renal-function tests are usually normal unless bladder neck and/or ureteral orifice obstruction has resulted in damage to the renal parenchyma from hydronephrosis or infection. An IVP is usually done to rule out a renal source of hematuria. During this procedure, the renal pelves are usually observed for the presence of a transitional cell carcinoma. At times such growths may present initially as a satellite lesion in the bladder. When cystograms are done, they usually demonstrate the location and scope of a filling defect in the bladder. Urinary cytology and ultraviolet cystoscopy following the administration of tetracycline are other diagnostic procedures which may be performed during the work-up of a patient suspected of having a bladder tumor.

The aforementioned cystoscopic technique is dependent upon the fluorescent properties of the tetracycline molecule. Some urologists believe this method is an especially useful means of locating cancerous areas within the bladder (Bowles, 1966).

THE TREATMENT OF BLADDER TUMORS

The main objectives in the care of the patient with a bladder tumor are the control of bleeding, the relief of pain, and the relief of dysuria. Before treatment is started, urinary dysfunction is usually corrected through the control of the infection. In some instances, chemotherapeutic agents are employed to accomplish this; in other cases, obstruction at the level of the ureter or vesical neck must be relieved. Since treatment depends on the size of the tumor and on the depth of its spread, the success of the course of treatment chosen as well as the prognosis for the patient are related to the histologic composition of the lesion. Superficial and early growths are often managed effectively by local surgical techniques accomplished with a resectoscope or through topical instillations of chemotherapeutic agents. Multiple lesions and infiltrating growths often require radical operation or radiation therapy. Thus the treatment of bladder tumors includes the topical administration of drugs, extensive or repeated endoscopic electroresections (transurethral resection) and fulguration, segmental resection of the bladder, or cystectomy. Radon seed implants are sometimes employed after endoscopic treatment. Irradiation is usually begun about a month after transurethral resection or any other surgical procedure. Currently, supervoltage irradiation has been of great benefit in the treatment of cancer of the bladder—especially when used in combination with surgical intervention. It has been found that the incidence of complications has been reduced as a result of this combined treatment modality.

Chemotherapeutic Methods of Treatment

Topical administrations of high concentrations of chemotherapeutic agents to the bladder are easily accomplished through a urethral catheter. When executing this treatment, the nurse should remember that the purpose of the instillation is to bathe the entire internal bladder mucosa with an antitumor drug. The most effective way of achieving this goal, therefore, is to insure that the patient is positioned so that the bladder tumor and the entire internal bladder wall come into contact with the solution being used. *Prior to the instillation of the drug*, the nurse should lower the head of the patient's bed to a position which is as flat as can be tolerated. During the bladder instillation, the patient should be advised to take slow, deep breaths. This tends to help him relax and thereby minimizes imagined discomforts of the treatment. After the drug has been introduced into the bladder, the patient should be instructed to alternate his position every 15 minutes. If the drug is to be retained for 1 hour the patient should lie flat on his back for 15 minutes, on his right side for 15 minutes, on his abdomen for 15 minutes, and finally on his left side for 15 minutes. If 2-hour retention is ordered, the cycle may be repeated again. Before the nurse leaves the bedside, a statement or two about the heightened effect of the treatment when the positional routine is followed usually reinforces the patient's motivation to cooperate. The call buzzer or call-light cord should always be placed within easy reach of the patient at this time so that he may summon the nurse if he experiences discomfort or any other difficulties during the treatment. The nurse should check the patient at 15-minute intervals during the course of the treatment to give words of encouragement and to reassure the patient that he has not been forgotten. Many patients fear that the nurse will "forget" to come back on time; others get discouraged because the time seems to pass so slowly.

5FU (5-fluorouracil) is an antimetabolite which has been administered topically in the treatment of bladder cancer. Usually, 10 mg per kilogram of body weight is dissolved in an equal volume of sterile water or saline for the weekly instillation of the drug. When administered as an adjunct to radiation therapy, it is believed that 5FU may act to potentiate the destructive effects of radiotherapy. However, it is known that absorption occurs from the bladder into the systemic circulation and a course of treatment with this drug may result in bone-marrow suppression. Then leukopenia may occur. Leukopenia is a reflection of bone-marrow suppression. Doctors usually keep a watchful eye on the patient's blood count throughout the duration of treatment. Toxicity to the drug is manifested by symptoms such as the loss of hair, moderate anorexia, nausea and vomiting, or melena (the passage of dark, pitchy, lumpy stools stained with blood pigments or with altered blood).

Weekly instillations of actinomycin D have also been administered topically. Actinomycin D is an antineoplastic antibiotic that has demonstrated suppressive activity against many experimental tumors. However, its value against human cancers is limited. When given, 1.0 mg of the drug is diluted with 30 ml of sterile water or saline.

Thio-TEPA is a multifunctional alkylating agent which has demonstrated favorable antitumor activity in man. It is effective on superficial tumors of the bladder mucosa—especially when generalized, diffuse lesions prohibit simple surgical resection. Thio-TEPA has also been used when patients with papillomatous growths are found to be poor surgical risks. Instillations of 30–60 mg of thio-TEPA in 30–60 ml of normal saline or sterile water have effected the complete disappearance of bladder tumors in some patients and the partial destruction of tumors in others. As few as seven instillations of this drug have accomplished these results. It is believed that the dosage mentioned may be retained for as long as 2 hours without resulting in a significant depressant effect on the bone marrow. Bone-marrow depression does occur, but within two to three weeks after administrations have been discontinued, the blood count returns within normal limits. A mild chemical cystitis is another toxic effect that has been noted in some patients.

Radiation Therapy

As previously stated, the control of bleeding and the relief of pain are primary objectives in the care of the patient with a bladder tumor. Clot formation occurs secondary to the bleeding, and clot retention secondary to obstructive processes often causes the patient to experience pain. Radiotherapy is sometimes used as a temporary means of controlling hemorrhage and for the relief of pain. However, such *palliative radiotherapy* is usually administered at dosages which are sublethal to the tumor. Many bladder tumors are radioresistant and, previously, such high dosages were necessary to arrest tumorous growths that contracture of the bladder and/or severe inflammation occurred. Today, however, supervoltage radiation is available for the treatment of such tumors.

A course of supervoltage radiation therapy usually begins with irradiation of the entire pelvis. If the individual's general health status is good or if he responds favorably to radiation therapy, a combination of radiation and surgical treatment may be employed. It has been demonstrated that a course of preoperative irradiation has diminished the incidence of postoperative complications in patients with bladder tumors. In a small percentage of cases, preoperative irradiation has even eradicated the bladder lesion. The rationale for the preoperative use of irradiation therapy is that this technique helps to contain infiltrating tumors locally within the bladder or in the pelvis. However, some urologists believe that when supervoltage radiation is used in the postoperative period it creates severe gastro-intestinal complications. Although the controversy continues, it is generally agreed that—when carefully managed—patients treated with supervoltage irradiation for bladder tumor tolerate the cancerocidal dosages well. Mild cases of diarrhea or proctitis have been reported and occasionally bright red bleeding secondary to rectal inflammation has also occurred. Most patients develop a transient episode of cystitis of varying intensity, but severe cystitis, bladder contraction, and ureteral or urethral stricture are not routinely encountered. When such complications are noted, it is believed that they occur most frequently because the course of radiation treatment was initiated too soon after a surgical procedure. Usually, radiation therapy is started no sooner than a month after such surgical procedures as transurethral resection, multiple biopsies with cauterization, suprapubic cystostomy, or segmental resection of the bladder.

High-energy radiation obtained from such sources as cobalt[60], the betatron, or the linear accelerator is under investigation as modalities for the primary treatment of advanced bladder cancer. However, the danger of severe rectal and bladder irritation secondary to these treatment sources is great.

The Resection of Bladder Tumors

Transurethral resection is the treatment of choice for patients with solitary or few papillary tumors located near the trigone area of the bladder. This method of treatment is recommended for small, superficial tumors which exhibit minimal tissue involvement. It is effective in curing many of the papillary carcinomas as well as the benign papillomas. Transurethral resection is accomplished with a resectoscope which is passed transurethrally. The objective of the surgeon's efforts is to fulgurate deeply enough into the bladder wall to remove the base of the tumorous growth. Cauterization of bleeders is accomplished concurrently, and gross bleeding is unusual. However, patients may complain of burning on urination subsequent to the treatment. Follow-up care consists of cystoscopic examination scheduled at regular intervals. Some urologists examine such patients every three months for the first year following operation and every six months thereafter. These tumors tend to recur either at the resection site or elsewhere in the body; therefore, follow-up cystoscopic examination is an essential part of the treatment plan.

Suprapubic electroresection of a bladder tumor is an open surgical procedure which is recommended when a bladder tumor cannot be treated adequately by transurethral resection. Electrical diathermy with or without radon seed implantation usually accomplishes this objective. The bladder is approached suprapubically and the base of the tumor as well as the surrounding tissue area is resected with an electrode-like instrument. When radon seed implantation is combined with this type of surgical resection, the seeds are placed (at equal distances from each other) into the area of the bladder from which the tumor was resected. Usual precautions of time, distance, and shielding should be observed by the nurse. A cystostomy tube may be left in place before closure of the bladder musculature has been completed, or a Foley catheter may be inserted to accomplish urinary drainage. The choice of drainage catheter usually depends upon the amount of bleeding present; a large cystostomy tube will facilitate the passage of clots if a significant amount of bleeding is present. The postoperative care is similar to that discussed for the patient following suprapubic cystostomy as treatment for the symptoms of prostatism (see Chapter 6).

Segmental resection of the bladder or *partial cystectomy* is the treatment of choice when superficial infiltration of the bladder musculature by tumor growth has occurred in the dome or mobile portion of the bladder. Utilization of this procedure is quite limited, however, because approximately 80 percent of the neoplastic growths of the bladder are located near the trigone region. Partial cystectomy has been employed for elderly patients with adenocarcinoma, transitional cell carcinoma, or squamous cell carcinoma when the lesion is well-defined, solitary, and inaccessible to adequate transurethral resection. Bimanual palpation of the empty bladder is an invaluable aid in helping the urologist evaluate the depth of tumor infiltration into the bladder musculature. Cystoscopy aids in a determination of the extent of surface area involved. Although involvement of the bladder neck precludes this method of treatment, involvement of one ureteral orifice is not a contraindication. An area of normal tissue surrounding the tumor mass must be present so that from 2 to 3 cm of that tissue may be excised along with the lesion. Therefore, only one ureteral orifice must be free of tumor. Multiple lesions grouped closely together may also be excised through this method. Either a transverse incision above the upper edge of the symphysis pubis or the usual suprapubic incision may be employed. The bladder is usually entered at a considerable distance from the site of the lesion and, after the area of resection has been defined, 2–3 cm of surrounding normal bladder wall are removed with the neoplasm. Ureteral reimplantation is sometimes necessary if the lesion is low in the bladder. After the resection has been completed, the bladder musculature is approximated and closure is started. If reimplantation of a ureter is indicated, it is done before insertion of the cystostomy tube and closure of the bladder. Penrose drains are usually placed perivesically and are brought out through the suprapubic opening. It should be mentioned that some risk of tumor implantation in the wound is present whenever a bladder containing a neoplasm is opened for surgical exploration.

The Penrose drains are usually advanced gradually for a three- to five-day interval before being removed. The cystostomy tube is allowed to drain the bladder for approximately

10 to 12 days. A urethral catheter is usually inserted when the cystostomy tube is withdrawn to enable more rapid closure of the suprapubic opening. By keeping the bladder empty, the urethral catheter aids in preventing the urine from oozing out of the suprapubic opening. Often, the patient will return to the unit with both catheters in place: a cystostomy tube and a urethral catheter. Many surgeons take this precaution to diminish the possibility of urinary retention from obstruction. Once the suprapubic tube has been removed and the opening has healed sufficiently, the urethral catheter is removed. The nurse may observe then that the patient voids frequently (sometimes as often as every 20 minutes) and in small amounts. The nurse should realize that the surgical procedure may reduce bladder capacity to as little as 60 ml. However, bladder tissue does regenerate to some extent and a capacity of from 200 to 400 ml may develop within a few months. The patient should be reassured, therefore, that his bladder capacity will increase over time and he should be encouraged to exercise patience. It may seem that the forcing of fluids is incompatible with this circumstance, but that assumption is erroneous. Fluid intake should be urged, but large quantities should be taken each time and the interval between fluid ingestion should be lengthened. This way the patient will not spend all of his waking time in or near the bathroom. To insure adequate rest during the night, fluids may be restricted after the dinner hour in the early evening. After being discharged from the hospital, visits to friends and/or other planned outings may be accomplished without undue embarrassment because of frequent trips to the bathroom. The nurse should instruct the patient to limit his fluid intake several hours prior to the time planned for leaving home. There will be adjustments to be made and inconveniences will be experienced during the first months after surgical intervention, but most patients regard this as a small price to pay for survival.

Cystectomy—the complete removal of the bladder—is indicated for those carcinomas which cannot be treated satisfactorily by transurethral resection, suprapubic electroresection, or partial cystectomy. This is the treatment of choice for deeply infiltrating types of carcinoma located near the trigone or at the bladder neck. It is also indicated for tumors which have demonstrated multiple recurrences and increasing cellular malignancy on biopsy. Generalized involvement of the bladder mucosa that cannot be controlled by other means is another indication for this procedure. However, cystectomy is usually not done when abdominal exploration demonstrates extravesical spread of the neoplasm with evidence of metastatic spread outside of the pelvis. The presence of positive pelvic lymph nodes also precludes utilization of this method. It has been reported that in some advanced cases an impressive degree of palliation has been obtained from the removal of the bladder. Thus cystectomy is sometimes used as the palliative treatment of choice even though usual practice would dictate only palliative urinary diversion in these cases *without* any surgical procedures being performed on the bladder itself.

Cystectomy involves the removal of the entire bladder; excised along with the bladder are the prostate gland, the seminal vesicles, and the perivesical fat. The patient is, of course, impotent postoperatively. When this procedure is utilized for the treatment of a female patient, the urethra and the uterus are also removed. It is generally agreed that radical lymph-node dissection is unnecessary, especially when the tumor has spread to the regional lymph nodes. This added radical procedure only tends to add to the morbidity and mortality resulting from such an operation. The prognosis is invariably poor if positive nodes are present. Once the bladder is removed, urine being propelled down the ureters must be expelled from the body through another route. Some method of permanent urinary diversion must be provided whenever cystectomy is performed. Nephrostomy, ureterostomy, or ureterointestinal anastomosis may be employed to divert the urinary stream. Some surgeons prefer to accomplish urinary diversion as a preliminary procedure. Others construct the diversion system in association with cystectomy. When the latter choice is made, the operative procedure is quite lengthy. Two approaches may be used to accomplish cystectomy: a combined perineal-abdominal approach or a suprapubic approach. The perineal-abdominal approach allows the prostate gland and base of the bladder to be freed from below, after which the rest of the bladder is liberated from above. If urinary diversion is combined with this procedure, the peritoneum must be entered. It is easily understood, therefore, why many surgeons prefer to manage the diversion of the ureters in a separate operation prior to cystectomy. Irradiation done after the construction of urinary diversion and before cystectomy often reduces the amount of bleeding from the tumor and provides relief of pain. Further, urinary diversion is usually safer before irradiation when renal damage, hydronephrosis, and/or infection is present. In the male patient, liberation of the prostate gland, seminal vesicles, and base of the bladder is hazardous because profuse bleeding is usually encountered. In the female patient, however, a vaginal approach accomplishes the separation of the base of the bladder from the vaginal wall and the uterus, which expedites the abdominal part of the procedure.

In the postoperative period, the patient requires intensive care. The bladder and large amounts of surrounding tissue are removed during the operation. If urinary diversion is done in association with cystectomy, the patient may have a stoma on the abdominal wall as well as a suprapubic incision and a perineal incision. The patient is kept NPO and receives intravenous fluids and electrolytes for several days. Replacement of blood loss is also important and the nurse should be certain that the patient has blood available on call. Vital signs are taken at frequent intervals for the first 48 to 72 hours. Observation of output is always crucial in the care of these patients and orders for the recording of the hourly amount of output is not unusual in the immediate postoperative period. Specific gravity determinations may be ordered every 4 hours. A nasogastric tube is usually in place because paralytic ileus is anticipated subsequent to the procedure. Dressings should be reinforced as needed. In developing the nursing-care plan, the nurse will have to integrate her knowledge of the essentials of care of the patient following abdominal surgery, care of the patient with a perineal incision, and care of the patient with the specific diversion system present. Priorities of care must be set if the plan is to be implemented successfully.

Cystectomy is no longer the debilitating operation that it used to be. In the past, diversion methods such as ureterostomy and ureterosigmoidostomy led to progressive renal failure and terminal uremia. Today, however, the ileal segment diversion system has provided encouraging results by lengthening the survival period. It has also been reported that the ileal conduit affords marked palliation for patients with *inoperable* bladder cancer. Such patients become extremely uncomfortable as the disease advances because of the local effects of the tumor and the hemorrhaging. Ileal segment diversion followed by irradiation has proved useful as palliative treatment for selected patients. For others, the objective of palliation may be the control of bladder infection with antibiotics or the removal of the kidney that is hydronephrotic and malfunctioning.

As stated earlier, diversion of the urinary stream must be provided for after cystectomy because the bladder is no longer available for the collection of the urine which flows down the ureters. Although urinary diversion may be indicated for congenital, traumatic, or severe inflammatory lesions of the bladder, it is most commonly performed because of carcinoma. Urinary diversion may be accomplished either through the surgical construction of a ureteral outlet on the skin surface (*an external ureteral diversion*) or through ureteral anastomosis to a section of intestine (*an internal ureteral diversion*).

EXTERNAL URINARY DIVERSION

There are two methods of surgical construction available to accomplish urinary diversion onto the skin surface: permanent nephrostomy and cutaneous ureterostomy. Construction of a permanent nephrostomy is usually a last-resort, life-saving measure that involves the insertion of a catheter through a subcostal incision in the flank. Through this procedure, a fistula is produced from the renal pelvis through the renal cortex. The catheter is usually held in position by a stay suture at each layer of closure. (The suture at the skin layer is removed approximately two weeks postoperatively and adhesive tabs retain the catheter afterwards.) The catheter is attached to gravity drainage and the urine drains into a collecting receptacle. Construction of a cutaneous ureterostomy involves the anastomosis of the ureters to the skin surface of the abdomen. An appliance positioned over the stoma collects the urine, which is constantly being discharged (see Fig. 3). Today, the continual use of catheters is generally avoided in cutaneous ureterostomies because they often aggravate strictures of the ureter and provide an avenue for infection. Stricture of the ureterostomy usually requires catheterization, however, unless a plastic procedure is performed on the anastomosis.

The Permanent Nephrostomy

The permanent nephrostomy is the least desirable of any of the urinary diversion procedures. The kidney and renal pelvis are exposed under direct vision through a subcostal flank incision and the upper ureter is ligated. A trocar is passed through the renal parenchyma into the renal pelvis with a stylet and, after the stylet has been withdrawn, a catheter is

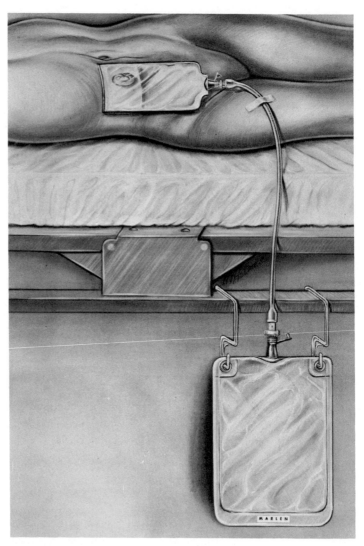

Fig. 3. Ureterostomy appliance positioned over the stoma. Drainage tubing is attached to a bedside gravity drainage set-up. The adherent part of this appliance may be adjusted to fit any sized stoma. It may be used temporarily during the postoperative period before the patient is fitted for an appliance sized especially for his ureterostomy. (Courtesy of the Marlen Mfg. & Development Co., Richmond Rd., Ohio.)

passed through the trocar into the renal pelvis. The trocar is then withdrawn from the parenchyma leaving the catheter in place. When the wound is closed, the catheter is brought out to the skin surface as straight as possible so that the pathway will allow easy removal and replacement during subsequent catheter changes. The catheter is then attached to straight gravity drainage. The incision is usually located as far anteriorly as possible to facilitate independent management of a drainage appliance when the patient is able to effect his own care. Surgeons also strive to construct the shortest tract possible between the skin surface and the renal pelvis. If direct visualization of the kidney is not possible, a "blind nephrostomy" is performed. This is accomplished from the outer curvature of the kidney by the insertion of an instrument through the renal cortex and into the renal pelvis. Then a self-retaining catheter may be introduced with a stylet. Regardless of the method used, the catheter is usually placed low in the kidney so that the lower calyx may be drained.

Although this procedure is easily accomplished, it must be remembered that the kidney parenchyma is highly vascular and that the potential for hemorrhage is great. Care is always taken during operation to avoid the disruption of vascular patterns within the kidney. Postoperatively, it should be remembered that the surgical procedures performed on the patient will cause him great discomfort and he will be inclined to resist turning, coughing, and deep breathing. Thus the danger of atelectasis and hypostatic pneumonia is great. Adequate medication for pain will enable the patient to accomplish the postoperative tasks which will prevent respiratory complications. It is a major nursing responsibility to insure that the patient is adequately medicated for pain. As pointed out earlier in this book, the fact that the patient has not asked for pain medication or appears to be sleeping restfully is no excuse for failure to administer medication during the early postoperative period. Rest is essential for recovery and this should be afforded the patient *between treatment intervals.* However, in order to accomplish the treatments, the patient must be relatively free of pain. Patients may appear "comfortable" because they have remained immobile for many hours—limiting motion so that the pain will be diminished.

The patient should not be allowed to remain flat on his back even though the nephrostomy tubes exit from both sides. As previously stated, the catheters will be situated as far anteriorly as possible and the nurse will find that a pillow bolster wedged under the back will maintain the patient in a position which is tilted toward the side. Meticulous care of the catheters and gravity drainage tubing is essential. When the patient is on bedrest, confusion is minimized if the catheters and tubing are allowed to drain *on the side of the bed closest to their exit site.* (In other words, the catheters and tubing draining the left kidney should be kept on the left side of the bed and those from the right kidney on the right side of the bed.) Repositioning of the patient may be accomplished by tilting him toward either side. It should be remembered that even when this is done, the nurse should make sure that the tubing from the left kidney is kept on the left side of the bed and vice versa. The patient should not lie on the tubing, however catheters tend to drain more efficiently when this is done, and movement will not cause entanglements or the pulling and tension that may lead to their dislocation. Patency of the tubing is vital to the patient's survival and the nurse should always check the tubing for twisting or kinking—especially after the patient's position is changed. Most doctors irrigate nephrostomy tubes only when absolutely necessary. However, when irrigations are ordered, sterile technique should be used whenever the catheters and open tubing are handled. Sterile normal saline is usually the solution of choice for irrigations, and the nurse should never allow more than 15 ml to enter the nephrostomy tube at any given time because of the limited capacity of the kidney pelvis. (In some cases hydronephrosis may have caused the enlargement of the renal pelvis to an extent that that structure is able to accommodate more solution. When this has occurred, the doctor usually indicates it on the order sheet.) During irrigations, complaints of cramplike pain are a warning to the nurse that too much solution has been introduced. However, if the catheter comes out, becomes plugged, or irrigates sluggishly, the irrigation should be discontinued and the doctor notified. Complaints of pain and/or chills should prompt the nurse to take the patient's temperature (to check for fever) and to notify the doctor. It should be noted that the doctor should be notified *immediately* whenever a catheter is dislodged because the lumen of the sinus tract contracts quickly and sometimes—even within a few hours—the tract may become obliterated and preclude insertion of another catheter. This eventuality would necessitate another operation. When the irrigation is completed, the amount of solution returned should be subtracted from the amount of solution used. Both the amount of solution used and the amount of solution retained within the pelvis should be recorded on the output sheet so that it may be subtracted from the actual urinary output. In this way, an accurate record of output is kept. A separate record must be kept for each catheter. The patient will also be receiving IV fluids; therefore, accurate intake as well as output records are essential.

Early ambulation is generally encouraged—depending on the overall condition of the patient—and leg urinals may be provided during waking hours, care being taken to avoid any pulling or tension on the nephrostomy tubes when the patient gets in and out of bed. The patient should be warned not to kink, twist, or lie on the tubing. The catheters are usually allowed to drain into bedside receptacles during the night. If a straight catheter is used, it is held in place with a stay suture (retention suture) for approximately two weeks postoperatively. Then the sutures are removed and adhesive tabs are used to hold the catheters at the exit site. This dressing should be changed every two or three days. Before the patient is discharged from the hospital, instruction regarding the daily care of nephrostomy tubes should be given to him and/or to the family member who will be carrying out his care at home. (Since nephrostomy-care routine varies from institution to institution, the hospital procedure book should be consulted by the nurse.) *Supervision while the patient is in the hospital* is very reassuring and should be continued periodically even after he exhibits competence with the procedures. Tub baths are usually allowed, but the patient should be told to remove the dressing before taking the bath. The adhesive tab securing the catheter usually becomes loosened during the bath and it will have to be reapplied. The dressing should also be replaced after the bath.

Some degree of infection is usually present in the majority of patients with permanent nephrostomies—even under optimal conditions. The catheters drain the kidney pelvis and, since their periodic replacement is necessary, the patient is predisposed to pyelonephritis. In some hospitals, nurses are allowed to change nephrostomy tubes, but this is usually a doctor's procedure. When the permanent nephrostomy drains are changed, the skin surrounding the catheter should be cleansed with PhisoHex and sterile water. The catheter should be clamped closed to the exit site on the skin surface so that a guide to the depth of insertion of the new catheter is provided. Prior to withdrawal of the catheter, the nurse should place a gloved hand firmly on the flank (near the tubing) so that support is afforded (see Fig. 4). Then, while the patient is taking a few deep breaths to aid in relaxtion, the catheter should be removed quickly. Subsequently, the same insertion distance should be measured off on the replacement catheter with another sterile clamp before it is introduced into the tract leading to the renal pelvis. The nurse must remember to keep the supportive hand firmly in place at the flank during the removal and replacement procedure. The tract is usually well established in these

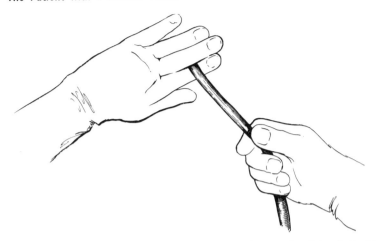

Fig. 4. Removal of a catheter from a nephrostomy. One gloved hand should be placed firmly at the flank over the nephrostomy tube.

patients and no difficulty will be encountered. In the manner described, the entire treatment may be accomplished within a few minutes. The catheter should be irrigated at this time with 5 to 10 ml of sterile saline and the returns allowed to flow into a sterile basin. The catheter will tend to fall at the patient's side in a natural position during this phase of the procedure and it may be secured with an adhesive tape tab thereafter. A new dressing applied around the nephrostomy tube over the exit site at the skin surface and connection of the tube to gravity drainage complete the treatment. The used catheters should be rolled between the palms of the hands before being washed with soap and water. This tends to loosen any encrusted salts within the lumen of the catheter; however, if salts and/or other accumulated material cannot be removed, the catheters must be discarded.

If catheter changes are performed in the home, rubber catheters may be soaked for 15 minutes in a solution of either vinegar and water (¼ cup vinegar in a quart of water) or household bleach and water (one teaspoon of bleach in one quart of water) to control odor. Subsequently, the catheters, irrigating bulb syringe or glass syringe, clamps, and basin should be rinsed with clear water. The catheters should be stored in a cool dry place. All equipment should be sterilized immediately before the next catheter change by being placed in a large strainer which is then lowered into a saucepan of water until the articles are covered by water. The equipment should be allowed to boil for 10 minutes after which time the strainer may be lifted out of the pan and the water discarded. Then the strainer may be replaced in the pan to permit cooling. Plastic catheters should be rinsed with water and allowed to dry thoroughly before being placed in a glass container and covered with a solution of aqueous zephiran 1:1000. Cold sterilization of plastic catheters is accomplished in 24 hours.

Cutaneous Ureterostomy

Ureterocutaneous anastomosis (cutaneous ureterostomy) is the urinary diversion procedure of choice when the patient's general physical condition precludes ureteral anastomosis that requires more extensive surgical methods. The primary goal of current surgical techniques is to fabricate a raised skin nipple in a location which permits urinary collection by a single device easily applied by the patient. Another goal is the prevention of ureteral constriction that would lead to urinary stasis and result in chronic pyelonephritis, renal calculi, and (eventually) renal failure. The stoma may be constructed either at the flank or on the anterior abdominal wall. However, even when divided close to the bladder, some degree of tension is exerted on the average ureter to enable it to reach the anterior abdominal wall. Therefore, for the past nine years, the high cutaneous ureterostomy (Berman, 1965) has gained popularity with surgeons. In this procedure, the upper half of the ureter is brought out to the skin by the shortest possible route. The stoma is constructed in the anterior axillary line about midway between the line of the twelfth rib and the iliac crest. Pressure, stretching, and kinking of the ureter is prevented because the ureter is allowed to remain in its normal retroperitoneal position. Earlier procedures utilized the distal third of the ureter and required the dissection of the ureter from its bed. The stoma was constructed on the anterior abdominal wall about halfway between the umbilicus and the anterior superior iliac spine.

Despite efforts to create an adequate skin nipple (or stoma), difficulty is continually reported. Sloughing of the distal ureteral stump, stenosis of the nipple, and excoriation of the skin secondary to urinary leakage frequently occur. Although it is generally agreed that the continual use of catheters in cutaneous ureterostomies should be avoided because of the possibility of pyelonephritis, the ureters are usually intubated with soft catheters in the early postoperative period to effect proper drainage of the renal pelvis. (The specifics of the important aspects of postoperative care of these patients are the same as those discussed in the preceding section.) The catheters remain in place for 10 to 14 days and a urinary collecting appliance is usually applied thereafter. When the collecting appliance is being used, a common complaint is the problem of achieving a watertight union between the skin and the urinary collecting appliance. Of major importance in this regard is the proper care of the skin surrounding the ureterostomy site and the proper application and removal of the ureterostomy appliance. The skin around the ureterostomy should be shaved with a safety razor as often as necessary. The circumference of the shaved area should be approximately 2 inches from the site of the stoma. A rolled gauze square should be held at the stomal opening to absorb urinary drainage from the stoma while the surrounding area is cleansed and allowed to dry. Then, tincture of benzoin should be applied to help toughen the skin and the area should be allowed to dry thoroughly once more. A thin coating of cement should then be spread evenly on the round disk or flange of the ureterostomy appliance which will come in contact with the skin surrounding the stoma. A thin coating of cement should also be spread on the skin. Fanning of the area will hasten the drying of the cement and contact between skin and appliance should be made only after the cement is dry. Urine flowing over the cement and onto the skin prior to the application of the device should be blotted up quickly with a dry section of the rolled gauze square. (Facial tissue rolled into a sausage-shaped blotter will also serve the purpose.) If a double-unit mounting ring and detachable cap device is used (the lip of the collecting device locks into a ring which remains mounted around the stoma), the mounting ring should be pressed firmly against the prepared skin area for about 5 minutes to ensure a watertight union. The cap may be snapped into place thereafter. Air pressure forming within the cap may be released by pulling one of the tabs on the cap until air escapes. If Sengers cups or another type of single-unit device is used (see Fig. 5), the lip or mounting ring of the device should be applied quickly over the ureterostomy with the opening centered over the stoma. Care should be taken to make sure that the drainage tubing is pointing downward. The ring should be held firmly against the skin for approximately 5 minutes to insure a good union. Once a good union has been established by either type of appliance, the drainage tubing should be attached to the urinary collecting receptacle (leg urinal during the day (see Fig. 6a, b); bedside collecting bottle at night, see Fig 7). For ease of carrying, a length of narrow cotton tape may be tied to the top of the leg urinal (through one of the openings available for the leg strap) and attached with a safety pin to an adhesive tape tab applied to the skin of the thigh a short distance above the urinal.

Removal and reapplication of either device should be done on a weekly basis. The best time for the change is usually in the morning upon rising. Since kidney function is lowest in the morning after an extended period of limited fluid intake,

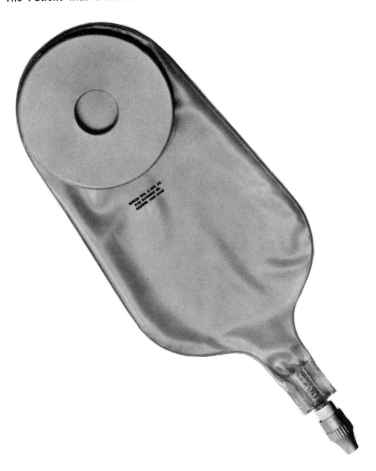

Fig. 5. A single-unit ureterostomy device. The flange (or mounting ring) visible at the top of the appliance is applied around the stoma. (Courtesy of the Marlen Mfg. & Development Co., Richmond Rd., Ohio.)

urinary drainage is minimal and leakage of urine over the freshly applied cement is less of a problem. For removal, the device should be gently peeled off like adhesive tape. A drop of benzine, acetone, or ether may be used on the edge of the mounting ring or disk to facilitate the process. It is not necessary to remove the cement from the disk at every change because

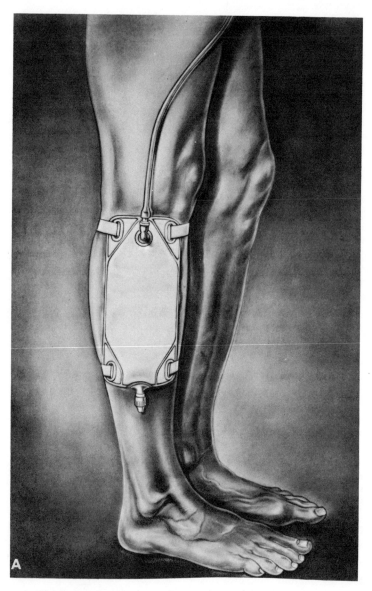

Fig. 6A. The ureterostomy drainage tubing attached to a leg urinal.

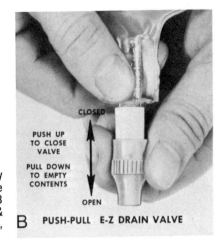

Fig. 6B. The urinal may be easily emptied by manipulation of the push-pull drain volve. (A and B Courtesy of the Marlen Mfg. & Development Co., Richmond Rd., Ohio.)

CLOSED

PUSH UP
TO CLOSE
VALVE

PULL DOWN
TO EMPTY
CONTENTS

OPEN

B   PUSH-PULL E-Z DRAIN VALVE

the roughened surface developed by accumulated layers of cement has a better sticking potential. *The cement should be peeled off*, however, when the coating reaches a thickness of about ⅛ inch. *Cement should be removed from the skin each time.* Rubbing with a finger or a gauze square will accomplish this task. Benzine may be used to aid in the process, but the nurse should remember to cleanse the area with alcohol and boric acid solution afterward so that skin irritation may be avoided. On the morning of the appliance change, the daily bath or shower should be taken during the interval between the removal of the soiled appliance and the application of the clean one.

The ureterostomy site should be carefully inspected at all times. Swollen or inflamed skin requires special care. Frequent warm baths with the appliance off should be followed by applications of tincture of benzoin to promote healing and toughening of the skin. It should be remembered that the peristaltic waves of the ureters move in a downward direction only so contamination of the tract by the bath water is not a

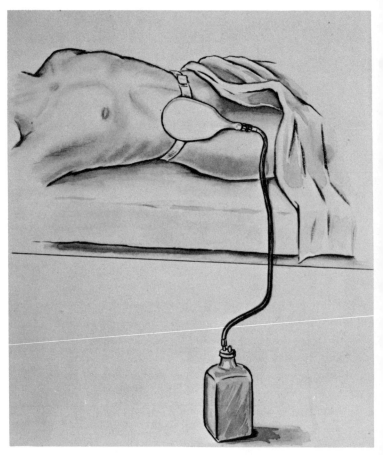

Fig. 7. The drainage tubing running from the ureterostomy appliance is attached to a bedside collecting bottle. (Courtesy of the Marlen Mfg. & Development Co., Richmond Rd., Ohio.)

problem. Local heat and air drying is the conservative treatment of choice for reddened and inflamed stomas.

Proper care of the appliance is also important, because adequate functioning depends on the treatment the appliance receives. The appliance should be washed with soap and water and rinsed thoroughly whenever changed. It should be allowed to air-dry in a cool place and care should be taken to hang the appliance so that no folds or kinks occur. Urinals should be changed and washed daily.

URETEROINTESTINAL ANASTOMOSIS

Review of the Anatomy and Physiology of the Intestinal Tract

The duodenum, the jejunum, and the ileum comprise the three sections of the small intestine (see Fig. 8). The duo-

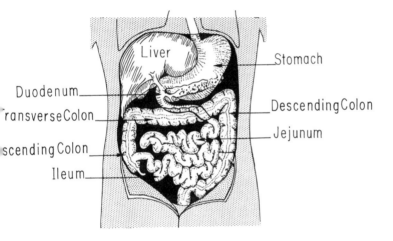

Fig. 8. The small and large intestine. (Redrawn from Dawson. Basic Human Anatomy. 1965. Courtesy of Appleton-Century-Crofts.)

denum is the shortest and widest part of the small intestine. The pyloric valve is located between the stomach and the duodenum. This first section of the small intestine is the only part that is anchored to the posterior abdominal wall. Of the other two remaining sections of the small intestine, the jejunum is thick-walled and more vascular than the ileal portion. It is shorter than the length of ileum, is situated centrally and in the lower part of the abdominal cavity, and the colon forms its superior and lateral boundaries. The ileum or last section of small intestine is continuous with the jejunum and terminates at the large intestine in the lower right quadrant of the abdomen. The ileocecal valve is located between this section of small intestine and the large intestine.

The jejunum and ileum are enclosed in the mesentery—a double layer of peritoneum which conveys blood vessels, lymphatics, and nerves to the intestinal tract. The mesentery attaches itself to areas of these two sections of small intestine in such a way that a regular series of loops is formed. The looping arrangement of the intestine discourages the formation of knots or twists along this elongated passageway. It is also the mesentery that loosely attaches the jejunum and ileum to the posterior abdominal wall. The anterior covering of the small intestine is provided by the greater omentum and the abdominal wall.

Nutrients are absorbed throughout the length of the small intestine by its walls. The mucosa, muscularis mucosa, and submucosal layers of the walls assume the shape of folds (or plicae) which project into the lumen of two sections of the small intestine: the jejunum and the ileum. The walls of the duodenum do not assume this shape. The folds are most pronounced in the jejunum and gradually diminish throughout the length of the ileum. They increase the absorption surface of the intestine. Small protuberances of the mucosal layer, called villi, are also present in the lumen of the small intestine. The majority are found in the duodenum and jejunum and may be seen on and between the plicae of these two sections. The villi also serve to increase the surface area available for the absorption of nutrients. It should be recalled at this juncture that most of the digestion and absorption of nutrients occurs in the small intestine.

The ileocecal valve at the distal end of the ileum marks the end of the small intestine and the beginning of the large intestine. Like the small intestine, the large intestine is also a continuous channel which is divided into numerous sections: the cecum, the colon (ascending, transverse, descending, and sigmoid), the rectum, and the anal canal. It can be distinguished from the small intestine because it is wider in appearance and the mucosa of its lumen contains no villi. However, there are numerous tubular, mucus-secreting glands within the walls of the lumen. The function of the ileocecal valve is to prevent the reflux of waste products from the *cecum*—an enlarged blind pouch situated in the lower right side of the abdominal cavity—back into the small intestine. This first part of the large intestine is continuous with the colon. When one is thinking of the names of the first three sections of the colon, it may be helpful to recall that they describe the direction followed by food residue as it travels through these segments of large intestine. The *ascending colon* rises upward from the lower right side of the abdominal cavity (see Fig. 8) and forms a lateral border for the small intestine. When the ascending colon reaches the level of the undersurface of the liver, it crosses the abdominal cavity and is therefore termed the *transverse colon*. After crossing the abdominal cavity, the colon descends along the left side of the cavity and this *descending section* of the *colon* eventually turns, curves, and terminates in the *sigmoid*. When at the midpelvic area, the sigmoid colon descends through the pelvis; it then becomes the *rectum*, and this last segment of large intestine ends at the *anus*.

The absorption of water is the primary function of the large intestine. Little absorption of nutritive material occurs within its lumen. After the food residue has passed from the small intestine into the large intestine, water is absorbed from the residue. The gradual dehydration that takes place results in the semisolid mass of feces which eventually reaches the rectum.

Surgical Procedures

As has been previously stated, when the bladder is totally removed (total cystectomy), some form of urinary diversion must be provided. If an internal method of diversion is chosen, the ureters may be anastomosed either to the intact intestine or to a segment of intestine which has been isolated from the main fecal stream. Although the ureters are occasionally anastomosed directly to the proximal urethra after total cystectomy, it should be noted that the urethral sphincter is of limited value when this operative procedure has been done. When an artificial bladder (a neobladder) is formed from a segment of bowel, however, it is attached to the prostatic urethra. This procedure has been utilized with some success, but poor emptying of the new bladder as well as residual urine have posed a problem. Even though the location of an anastomosis of the ureters may vary, the fundamental concept underlying the implantation of the ureters when total cystectomy has been performed is that the site chosen should permit unobstructed drainage of urine away from the kidney, continent storage of urine, minimum absorption of urinary matter, and relative freedom from infection.

A serious complication which may arise from the diversion of urine into the bowel is *hyperchloremic acidosis*. Since more chloride ions than sodium ions are absorbed into the bloodstream from the colon, an imbalance of blood electrolytes tends to occur when the bowel is exposed to urine. It should be evident then that the degree of absorption is directly related to the surface area of bowel involved. Thus, in principle, more absorption occurs when the ureters are anastomosed to the intact bowel because the entire large intestine is exposed to urine. Conversely, a small, isolated loop of bowel used as a conduit (passageway) for urine would allow less absorption of the constituents that cause hyperchloremic acidosis. In addition to the surface area exposed to urine, factors such as the segment of bowel involved and the frequency of emptying of the bowel play an important role in the development of electrolyte imbalance in the patient with urinary diversion into intact bowel. Bicarbonate concentration is higher and chloride content is lower in the colon than in the plasma, disturbance of the acid-base balance in the body is usually related to the exchange of the ions of those substances in association with the production and absorption of ammonia. It is generally agreed that—to a great degree—normal kidneys can correct such an imbalance when it occurs; however, if any degree of obstruction or infection is present, this ability may become greatly impaired. Therefore, another factor which may contribute to the development of electrolyte imbalance is the functional capacity of the kidney; and it may be concluded that acidosis may occur as a result of absorption from the colon, from functional impairment which may alter the tubular base-sparing mechanism of the kidney, or from a combination of the two.

Many surgeons and patients prefer ureterointestinal anastomosis to external methods of urinary diversion because of the negative aspects of constantly draining urine. However, the belief that accumulated urine in the bowel predisposes to disturbances of body chemistry is a strong deterrent to the utilization of this method by many other surgeons. Advocates of the ureterointestinal anastomosis counter that when ureteral obstruction, renal impairment, or reflux resulting in pyelonephritis is absent, the incidence of body chemistry disequilibrium is negligible.

Today, antibiotics and other chemotherapeutic agents permit adequate cleansing and sterilization of the bowel in preparation for operation as well as prophylactic treatment during the postoperative period. Further, the technical success of the procedure depends on an anastomosis that will not constrict. Therefore the elimination or attenuation of infection prior to and following surgical intervention aids in the reduction of the incidence of stricture and tissue breakdown at the site of the implantation of the ureters into the bowel.

A low-residue diet is usually ordered for the patient for a period of three to four days preoperatively. Some surgeons regress the diet during this period so that the diet restriction goes from low-residue to liquids to nothing by mouth. Administrations of neomycin and/or sulfathalidine to sterilize the bowel are usually given for approximately 48 hours prior to operation. *Cleansing enemas until clear returns are obtained* are given prior to and during the evening before the procedure, as needed. To assist the patient in adjusting to the feeling of fluid in the bowel—if the ureters are to be implanted into intact bowel—the nurse should allow approximately 300 ml of the enema solution to flow in at a time and instruct the patient to retain the solution as long as possible before expelling it. During the preoperative interval, the nurse should further prepare the patient about what to expect in the postoperative period. It should be explained that he will receive IV fluids during the initial postoperative days. He should also be told that a nasogastric tube will be in place. It is important to give the patient —and his family, whenever possible—a simple explanation of the reason for the postoperative procedures so that maximum cooperation may be obtained. The importance of coughing and deep breathing should also be stressed, and practice ventilation exercises should be done for brief periods daily. Patients often "forget" how to accomplish this task after the operation and it will be necessary to repeat the instructions and to lend emotional support in most instances. The student should remember that the purpose of the preoperative instruction is primarily to prepare the patient for what he should anticipate in the postoperative period, so that emotionally he may begin to deal with the forthcoming situation and with what will be expected of him.

Ureterosigmoidostomy

The suffix -*ostomy* indicates an "opening into"; when ureterosigmoidostomy is performed, the ureters are implanted into the sigmoid section of the intact bowel so that urine flows into the sigmoid—which acts as a reservoir (see Fig. 9). Postoperatively, urinary output must be carefully measured because urinary suppression may occur. Anuria will be noted if this happens. When anuria occurs following ureterosigmoidostomy, it seldom exceeds a 24-hour period. Usually, constant drainage of the diversion site is effected by a large rectal tube that remains in place until the tenth postoperative day. The tube is usually inserted approximately 4 inches into the rectum and taped to the buttock to secure it in place. If for any reason the rectal tube should become obstructed, the doctor should be notified so that he may change it. *The nurse should not change the rectal tube in the early postoperative period* because of the danger of tissue perforation around the site of the ureteral anastomosis. A nasogastric tube will also be in place and the patient will be receiving IV fluids. Nursing responsibility for the accurate recording of intake and output should be stressed. When audible bowel sounds are noted, the nasogastric tube is removed and the patient's diet is gradually progressed from fluids to low-residue to a regular diet. During this interval, the rectal tube may be removed by the nurse when the patient has the desire to defecate. After defecation, the rectal tube may be replaced by the nurse, but it must be remembered that the tube should be inserted into the rectum *no more than 4 inches*. This length should be measured off and a strip of adhesive should be taped around the tube as a marker prior to insertion. After the period of frequent measurement of urinary output has passed, the rectal tube is usually removed during the day and replaced only at night. The rectal sphincter insures continence

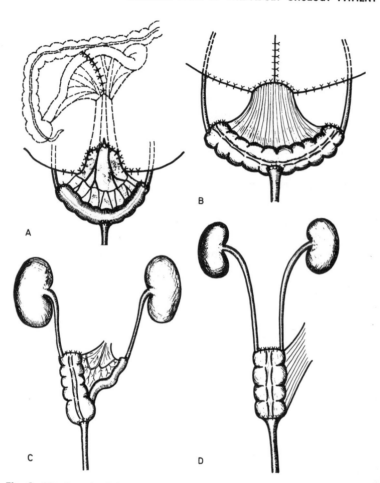

Fig. 9. Attachment of isolated intestinal segments to the urinary tract with implantation of both ureters and anastomosis to the urethra. A. An ileal segment. B. A sigmoid segment. C. A U-shaped ileocecal segment. D. An I-shaped sigmoid segment. (From Hardec. **J. Urol.**, 94:407, 1965. Courtesy of The Williams & Wilkins Co.)

during the waking hours, but nocturnal enuresis often proves a problem when the patient is asleep. The reinsertion of the tube at night, therefore, insures adequate urinary drainage as well as adequate rest for the patient.

While the diet is being progressed, diarrhealike bowel movements may be distressing to the patient. He should be reassured that this is to be expected during that period in which the bowel is adjusting to the presence of urine. As the bowel adjusts, a soft stool will be characteristic. Eventually however, the patient will be able to differentiate between the urge to defecate and the urge to urinate. Often as much as 200 ml of urine may be retained by the sigmoid reservoir before the patient feels the urge to urinate.

Prior to the day when the patient is discharged from the hospital, the nurse should prepare him for independent self-care. The important modifications of behavior that will be essential to his subsistence should be stressed. Unless the doctor orders a special diet for the patient, a regular diet may be permitted and the nurse should encourage the patient to continue drinking 3,000 ml (or 15 glasses of fluid) daily after discharge from the hospital. Fifteen glasses is an imposing number to most patients and, although few achieve this task, adequate hydration is usually accomplished by the time the patient has finished the equivalent of 10 glasses. Most of the patients are placed on maintenance dosages of drugs as a preventive measure against infection in the upper urinary tract, but an essential adjunct to the drug therapy is adequate fluid intake to insure what may be called the *natural* or *physiologic irrigation* of the kidney pelvis and ureters. The patient should also be advised to retain urine no longer than 4 hours. He should void every 3 to 4 hours while awake, and should insert a rectal tube at bedtime. A simple explanation may be given about the absorptive characteristic of the bowel. Thereafter he may better understand why the frequent emptying of urine from the bowel is essential to prevent the reabsorption of waste products which the body has discarded into the urine. It should also be explained that frequent evacuation of the bowel tends to improve the emptying of the ureters and renal pelvis. During such a discussion of the reabsorption of waste products from the bowel, the nurse should take advantage of the opportunity to inform the patient about the symptoms of electrolyte imbalance. The patient should be told to call the doctor immediately if he experiences prolonged periods of nausea, vomiting, diarrhea, or lethargy. Instruction regarding the insertion of the rectal tube at bedtime should also be given. A demonstration of the taping of the tube at the 4 inch length from the tip should be given. Practice insertions should they be done until the patient feels competent to perform the procedure without supervision. Since the rectal tube will be connected to a gravity drainage system, the patient should be taught how to cleanse the tubing so that odor may be controlled. An inexpensive way to deodorize the tubing is to soak it for 15 minutes in white vinegar after it has been thoroughly washed through with soap and water and rinsed with clear water. Cold sterilization solution may be obtained in economic quantities at the medical supply stores where the rectal tubes and drainage tubing are sold. The patient should be told that the rectal tube must be *clean* before insertion; sterile technique is unnecessary. A special word of caution should be given about the taking of enemas and strong cathartics because both cause peristalsis in the lower bowel to increase. Such an increase might force urine contaminated with fecal contents into the ureters and initiate an infection. Finally, at the time of discharge, the nurse should advise the patient that if for some other reason he is readmitted to a hospital, he or a member of his family or some identification-type card he carries should tell the staff that he voids through his rectum.

Most of the criteria for the free drainage of urine away from the kidney are met by the ureterosigmoidostomy method of urinary diversion. The operation is not as difficult or time-consuming as other diversionary methods, the problem of maintaining the blood supply to an isolated loop of bowel is averted, and—because ultimately the rectosigmoid reservoir can retain as much as 400 ml of urine—one can void without *undue* frequency. The anal sphincter is utilized to control both urine and feces; in most cases, the normal tone of this sphincter insures continence during the waking hours. Thus it would seem that implantation of the ureters into a sigmoid reservoir would be a nearly ideal site for urinary diversion. However, two problems are commonly encountered following this procedure: frequent episodes of pyelonephritis and, subsequently, renal insufficiency. Nephrolithiasis has also occurred.

Although urinary drainage away from the kidney is effected, renal function is not preserved. A predisposition of the patient to infection is inherent in this method. It should be remembered that pressure within the rectum is higher than bladder pressure. (Normally, more pressure is exerted when an individual is defecating than when he is urinating.) After cystectomy is performed and the ureters are implanted into the sigmoid section of the colon, a relatively higher pressure gradient exists between the colon and the ureters. Therefore, when waste products (fecal or urinary) are being evacuated from the colon, fecal contents may be forced upward into the ureters and kidney pelvis. A significant incidence of *fecal reflux* has been noted and infection—usually pyelonephritis—inevitably leads to uremia, which causes death. In addition to the possibility of infection, predisposition to electrolyte imbalance is also inherent in this method of urinary diversion. As previously stated, absorption is a primary function of the intestinal tract. Urinary waste products—especially chlorides—may be reabsorbed, with hyperchloremic acidosis resulting. When this occurs, the acid-base balance of the body may be reestablished through diet, administrations of sodium bicarbonate and/or alkalizing agents, and by encouraging frequent evacuation of waste from the bowel. However, in instances in which these measures do not correct hyperchloremic acidosis, further surgical procedures can be employed to convert the diversion of urine into a rectosigmoid bladder after a proximal colostomy has been performed. Generally speaking, the results from ureterosigmoidostomy have been disappointing and this method is usually employed for the patient with a relatively short life expectancy.

Ileal Conduit

A *conduit* is a passageway or channel through which water is conveyed. Unlike the reservoir type of diversionary procedure, the conduit acts only as a passageway through which urine may be propelled and eliminated; storage of urine is not effected. The ileal conduit represents the anastomosis of the ureters to an *isolated section* of intestine which is subsequently constructed into an ileostomy (see Fig. 10). An ileal

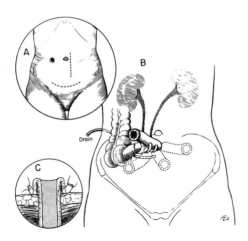

Fig. 10. Operative technique for ureteroileal anastomosis. (From **Clin. Obstet. Gynec.**, 8:726–756, 1965. Courtesy of Dr. William Scott.)

segment is suitable for urinary diversion because of its accessibility and peristaltic activity. It will permit the urine to be expelled from the body by peristalsis. To accomplish the operation, a segment of ileum (an ileal loop) about 6 inches from the ileocecal valve is often used. The loop and its mesentery—

containing the blood supply—are isolated from the rest of the intestine and the severed ends of intestine are reanastomosed, thereby leaving the intestinal tract rejoined and continuous once more. Thereafter, one end of the ileal segment is closed and the ureters are anastomosed to the wall of that segment near the closed end. The distal or open end of the loop is everted at a preselected site on the skin surface and sutured to the skin to form the external stoma of the ileostomy. Internally, the loop is secured to the peritoneum; then the abdomen is closed. During the procedure, care is always taken to preserve the correct peristaltic direction of the ileal segment so that urine entering the segment from the ureters will be conveyed toward the ileostomy opening and into a urinary collecting appliance.

Postoperatively, a temporary ileostomy bag is carefully applied over the stoma. Urinary output is measured at 2-hour intervals (or more frequently if indicated) for as long as necessary. Catheters are seldom inserted into the ileal segment. In the early postoperative period, it will be noted that the ileal segment will empty more completely when the patient is lying in the supine position or on his right side. However, after the blood pressure has stabilized, a semi-Fowler, or sitting position may be permitted. The nurse should remember to check the bag for twisting and kinking when the patient's position is being changed.

Intravenous fluids are given and a nasogastric tube is kept in place until effective intestinal peristalsis has returned. Gastric suction is usually ordered and the patient is allowed nothing by mouth until the site of the ileal anastomosis has healed. In a few days, the nasogastric tube will be clamped for 24 hours while oral intake is progressed to clear fluids (often 30 ml per hour initially). Intravenous administrations of fluids are continued during this time. When bowel sounds return and no distention or vomiting occurs, the nasogastric tube is removed. Diet is progressed from full fluids to soft diet to diet, as tolerated.

Early ambulation is the general rule for these patients. It serves the threefold purpose of helping to prevent postoperative respiratory complications, improving urinary evacuation through the conduit, and raising the morale of the patient. The ileostomy bag should be changed periodically to prevent odor and to protect the skin. When the bag is removed, the area surrounding the ileostomy stoma should be cleansed with acetone to remove any remnants of adhesive substance remaining on the skin. Tincture of benzoin applied to the skin area thereafter (prior to the placement of the new temporary bag) is of help in providing the skin with a protective coating and in encouraging the new bag to stick securely. Approximately two weeks after surgery, abdominal distention and edema of the stoma has subsided sufficiently to permit measurement of the patient for his permanent ileostomy appliance.

A good fit is obtained if the appliance completely covers the skin without rimming or crowning of the ileal stoma. It should be remembered, however, that it takes about a month for the stoma to shrink to its permanent size. At one time patients were taught to dilate the stoma by inserting a finger (covered with a finger cot and well lubricated) through the stoma opening daily for a time and then on a weekly basis. Today, however, the surgical technique has been refined and the ileal stomas are so meticulously formed that fingering of the stoma is unnecessary.

About two weeks after the operation, a flat plate of the abdomen and an IVP are done in order to check the length, dilatation, and degree of ileoureteral reflux present. (This is usually repeated in six months.) Then, before the patient is discharged, catheterization of the ileal segment through the ileal stoma (cleansed prior to the procedure) is usually done so that urine sample for culture and sensitivity may be obtained. During the course of the catheterization, the emptying efficiency of the ileal segment may be ascertained from the amount of residual urine present in the conduit. If the culture yields a significant bacterial count, appropriate drug therapy is given. Catheterization is usually repeated either during follow-up visits or annually. Intravenous urograms are also given on an annual or biennial follow-up basis.

Before discharge from the hospital, the importance of keeping follow-up appointments should be stressed. Weekly or more frequent periodic removal and replacement of the ileostomy appliance should also be stressed. The patient should be allowed sufficient time for supervised practice applications prior to discharge Any questions about cleansing of the appliance and/or personal hygiene should be answered at this time. (Information pertaining to these concerns is included in the discussion of ureterostomies.)

As noted earlier, it is the area of mucosal surface exposed to urine that is primary to the development of hyperchloremic acidosis. The active peristaltic action within the conduit, together with the low intraluminal pressure and the relatively empty state of that short ileal segment, preclude a high incidence of hyperchloremic acidosis. It should be remembered, however, that the peristaltic movements of the conduit rarely accomplish complete emptying of the channel. Usually only small spurts of urine are propelled from the blind end of the conduit to the exterior. Therefore, the conduit will always be found to retain varying amounts of urine. However, when acidosis does follow an ileac diversion of this kind, it is usually attributed to preexisting renal disease.

Radiologic observation via retrograde cinefluorography has demonstrated a lack of coordination between ureteral and conduit contractions. Sudden episodes of massive reflux have been observed after ureteral contractions, especially when a subsequent conduit contraction occurred near the site of the ureteroileal anastomosis. Thus, it can be understood why these patients are predisposed to hydronephrosis. Urine cultures from the conduits often yield significant pathogenic bacterial counts. Although complications such as pyelonephritis and renal insufficiency may occur, recurrent pyelonephritis with uremia occurs infrequently. Ileal conduits have many advantages over methods of anastomosis to intact bowel. With the ileal conduit there is no fecal contamination, minimal stasis of urine, no reabsorption of waste products, no sphincter dependence, no inherent predisposition to infection, and freedom from nightly catheter insertions. However, many serious complications have been reported. The possibility of peritonitis, intestinal obstruction, wound sepsis, and urinary leakage from the blind end of the conduit is great. There have also been incidents of elongation and malfunction of the ileal segment secondary to distal obstruction of the loop. Stomal complications are no longer as frequent a problem since the development of improved surgical techniques for construction of these areas, as well as the implementation of more diligent postoperative care. Today, surgeons strive to construct a "rose bud" nipple which will easily admit a finger and make dilation unnecessary. The stoma is usually constructed near the belt line because this is a site well suited for comfortable placement of the urinary collecting appliance. In the postoperative period, folded sponges should be placed around the part of the temporary drainage bag which surrounds the stoma so that leakage of urine onto the skin will be prevented. The patient is usually fitted for a suitable appliance as soon as possible because repeated removal and reapplication of temporary bags often causes damage to the skin surrounding the stoma. The importance of a properly fitting appliance should be stressed at this juncture. Chronic irritation leading to keratosis, ulceration, maceration, and even hemorrhage of the stomal mucosa may result from an appliance which is either tight or too freely movable. Further, the pooling of urine in a poorly fitted appliance predisposes the patient to infection. A quick-drying cement is recommended for placement of the appliance, and *it should be applied in a thin film* on both the disk or mounting ring of the appliance (the circular band which comes in contact with the skin surrounding the stoma) and the skin around the stoma. The nurse should make sure that both surfaces are dry—*not tacky*—before contact is established. Approximately three to five minutes after the cement has been applied, the nurse may touch the cement to ascertain the degree of dryness. This precaution is important because air bubbles often become trapped when contact of tacky surfaces is established. These bubbles undermine the water-tightness of the appliance. Urine escapes under the ring onto the skin, and maceration may result. The nursing-care plan should allow sufficient time for instructing the patient in order to insure his competence and confidence with a new device. The patient should also be advised that skin ulceration may be treated with the application of local heat and air-drying, this can easily be accomplished at home by using a portable ladies' hairdryer. After the skin has healed, applications of tincture of benzoin are often useful to toughen the skin. The importance of keeping follow-up appointments should always be stressed prior to the patient's discharge from the hospital.

Although many surgeons agree that the conduit procedure is superior to all other methods of ureterointestinal anastomosis, patients find it less acceptable than procedures which utilize urethral or anal orifices of elimination. Dependence on an external urinary appliance is considered a disadvantage by patients. Further, skin irritation near the stoma may become complicated by a *Monilia* infection and cause great discomfort for the patient.

Other Ureterointestinal Diversion Procedures

The *wet colostomy* represents the anastomosis of the ureters to the colon at a site above a colostomy. The ureters are anastomosed close to the colostomy stoma (usually no more than 4 to 5 inches proximal to the stoma). The length of time

needed to accomplish this procedure is relatively short and—
in patients who already have a colostomy—construction of a
second stoma is avoided. The primary disadvantages of this
procedure are the intrinsic danger of infection to the urinary
tract and the control of odor. Although hyperchloremic acidosis
occurs infrequently, it does occur.

The *rectal bladder* is currently the procedure of choice
for many surgeons when the patient has a life expectancy of
10 years or more. When the objectives of a urinary diversion
method are reviewed, it will be noted that the objective of keeping the urine separate from fecal contents is achieved because
a segment of rectum is isolated and an abdominal colostomy
is furnished. The ureters are anastomosed to the isolated rectal
segment after a terminal sigmoidostomy has been constructed.
The anal sphincter provides continence during the day and a
small rectal tube may be inserted to prevent leakage during
the night. The objective of maintaining renal function is
achieved because ascending urinary infection is reported infrequently. Usual colostomy care and application of a clean
compress are the only requirements for the maintenance of the
dry colostomy. An advantage of this procedure is that a collecting apparatus on the abdomen is not needed. Electrolyte
imbalance is seldom noted because there is a smaller mucosal
surface available for the absorption of urinary elements. Morbidity is negligible.

A section of sigmoid large enough to form a new bladder
or neobladder is sometimes isolated to accomplish urinary diversion. The ureters are joined to the isolated segment and the
sigmoid is anastomosed directly to the posterior urethra. After
a certain amount of urine has accumulated within the sigmoid
reservoir, the internal pressure leads to a sensation of the urge
to urinate. The voluntary evacuation of the neobladder is
mediated via the external sphincter. The construction of a neobladder is rarely done following total cystectomy for carcinoma
because it necessitates allowing a portion of urethra and pros-

tate gland (that portion which includes the external urinary sphincter) to remain—although it should be removed as part of the total resection. Another objection to the procedure is that a larger surface area of intestine is exposed to urine, and this predisposes the patient to electrolyte imbalance.

Most urologists agree that—of all the ureterointestinal techniques employed—the ileal conduit is best for urinary diversion. The conduit procedure is employed after cystectomy for the cure of bladder cancer and for many neurogenic and congenital conditions. It has also been used as a palliative procedure for the elimination or reduction of bleeding, for ureteral obstruction, and for dysuria and pelvic pain when resection of the primary tumor was not possible. Further, the conduit procedure has been utilized preliminary to the implementation of chemotherapy and/or irradiation therapy in the treatment of bladder tumors. However, despite technical improvements in the performance of the procedure and fewer reports of postoperative complications, patients continue to exhibit varying degrees of weakness, fatigue, anorexia, nausea and vomiting, diarrhea, and dehydration. These symptoms have been noted in patients during an interval of from one to several years following surgical intervention, and even death may occur. The preexisting disease process which necessitated the construction of the diversion system is considered to be the cause of these unfortunate complications.

REFERENCES

1. Berman, H. I. Urinary diversion in treatment of carcinoma of bladder. Surg. Clin. N. Amer., 45:1495–1508, 1965.
2. Bloedorn, F. G., et al. Radiotherapy in the treatment of cancer of the bladder. Southern Med. J., 60:539–544, 1967.
3. Bowles, W. T. Carcinoma of the urinary bladder. Med. Times, 94:735–739, 1966.

4. Campbell, J. E., et al. Dynamics of ileal conduits. Radiology, 85:338–342, 1965.
5. Cardonnier, J. J. Cystectomy in the management of carcinoma of the urinary bladder. Postgrad. Med. J., 41:469–470, 1965.
6. Dawson, H. L. Basic Human Anatomy. New York, Appleton-Century-Crofts, 1966, pp. 210–216.
7. Dick, V. S., and Zinman, L. Partial Cystectomy with ureteral reimplantation in the treatment of bladder neoplasm. Surg. Clin. N. Amer., 45:723–727, 1965.
8. Dowd, J. B., and Shah, S. Technique of uretero-ileal-cutaneous anastomosis ("the ileal loop"). Surg. Clin. N. Amer., 45:741–750, 1965.
9. Esquivel, E. L., et al. Treatment of bladder tumors by instillation of thio-TEPA, actinomycin D, in 5-fluorouracil. Invest. Urol., 2:381–386, 1965.
10. Early diagnosis of bladder cancer. Brit. Med. J., 1:253–254, 1967.
11. Frenay, M. A. C., Sr. A dynamic approach to the ileal conduit patient. Amer. J. Nurs., 64:80–83, 1964.
12. Furlow, W. L., and Mussey, E. The "silent" vesical neoplasm. J.A.M.A., 204:76–77, 1968.
13. Glantz, G. M. Cystectomy and urinary diversion. J. Urol., 96:714–717, 1966.
14. Gonick, P., et al. Stage B carcinoma of the bladder: Treatment and results in 71 cases. J. Urol., 99:728–732, 1968.
15. Hanley, H. G. Urinary diversion in carcinoma of the bladder. London Clin. Med. J., 7:49–55, 1966.
16. Higgins, R. B. Bilateral transperitoneal umbilical ureterostomy. J. Urol., 92:289–294, 1964.
17. Home Care for the Patient After Urological Surgery. Nursing Division, Memorial Hospital of Cancer and Allied Diseases (Treatment Unit of Memorial Sloan-Kettering Cancer Center).
18. Jewett, H. J. Tumors of the bladder. In Campbell, M. F., ed. Urology, 2nd ed. Philadelphia, W. B. Saunders Company, 1963, Vol. 2, pp. 1027–1096.
19. Laskowski, T. Z., et al. Combined therapy: Radiation and surgery in the treatment of bladder cancer. J. Urol., 99:733–739, 1968.
20. Markland, C., and Flocks, R. H. The ileal conduit stoma. J. Urol., 95:344–349, 1966.
21. Massey, B. D., et al. Carcinoma of the bladder: 20-year experience in private practice. J. Urol., 93:212–216, 1965.
22. Mount., B. M., et al. Ureteral implantation into ileal conduits. J. Urol., 100:605–609, 1968.
23. Newman, D. M., et al. Squamous cell carcinoma of the bladder. J. Urol., 100:470–473, 1968.

24. Scott, W. W. Methods of urinary diversion in radical pelvic surgery. Clin. Obstet. Gynec., 8:726–756, 1965.

25. Symmonds, R. E. Use of the colon for urinary diversion. Clin. Obstet. Gynec., 10:217–226, 1967.

26. Tollefson, D. M. Nursing care of the patient with an ileac diversion of the urine. Amer. J. Nurs., 59:534–536, 1959.

27. Veenema, R. J., et al. Bladder carcinoma treated by direct instillation of thio-TEPA. J. Urol., 88:60–63, 1962.

28. Walsh, M. A., et al. Neobladder. Amer. J. Nurs., 63:107–110, 1963.

29. Woodruff, M. W., et al. Further observations on the use of combination 5-fluorouracil and supervoltage irradiation therapy in the treatment of advanced carcinoma of the bladder. J. Urol., 90:747–758, 1963.

30. Yonometo, R. H., et al. Evaluation of ileal conduit as a palliative procedure. Surg. Gynec. Obstet., 121:70–78, 1965.

Index